Endocrinology at a Glance

Endocrinology at a Glance

BEN GREENSTEIN
Arizona Arthritis Center
College of Medicine
University of Arizona
Tucson, AZ 85724-5093
USA

Blackwell
Science

Blackwell Publishing Company
Editorial Offices:
9600 Garsington Road, Oxford OX4 2DQ.
23 Ainslie Place, Edinburgh EH3 6AJ
350 Main Street, Malden
MA 02148 5018, USA
54 University Street, Carlton
Victoria 3053, Australia
10, rue Casimir Delavigne
75006 Paris, France

Other Editorial Offices:
Blackwell Wissenschafts-Verlag GmbH
Kurfürstendamm 57
10707 Berlin, Germany

Blackwell Science KK
MG Kodenmacho Building
7-10 Kodenmacho Nihombashi
Chuo-ku, Tokyo 104, Japan

Iowa State University Press
A Blackwell Science Company
2121 S. State Avenue
Ames, Iowa 50014-8300, USA

First published 1994
Four Dragons edition 1994
Reprinted 1996, 1998, 2001, 2002, 2004

Set by Setrite Typesetters, Hong Kong
Printed and bound in India by Thomson Press (I) Ltd.

For further information on
Blackwell Science, visit our website:
www.blackwellpublishing.com

DISTRIBUTORS

Marston Book Services Ltd.
PO Box 269
Abingdon
Oxon OX14 4YN
(*Orders:* Tel: 01235 465500
Fax: 01235 465555)

The Americas
Blackwell Publishing
c/o AIDC
PO Box 20
50 Winter Sport Lane
Williston, VT 05495-0020
(*Orders:* Tel: 800 216 2522
Fax: 802 864 7626)

Australia
Blackwell Science Pty Ltd
54 University Street
Carlton, Victoria 3053
(*Orders:* Tel: 3 9347 0300
Fax: 3 9347 5001)

A catalogue record for this title
is available from the British Library

ISBN 0-632-03835-7 (BSP)
ISBN 0-632-03837-3 (Four Dragons)

Library of Congress
Cataloging in Publication Data

Greenstein, Ben, 1941
Endocrinology at a glance/Ben Greenstein.
p. cm.
Includes bibliographical references
and index.
ISBN 0-632-03835-7 (BSP ed.)
ISBN 0-632-03837-3 (4 Dragon ed.)
1. Endocrinology, 1. Title.
[DNLM: 1. Endocrine Glands. 2. Hormones,
WK 100 G815e 1994]
QP187.G834 1994

Contents

Introduction

Endocrinology at a Glance is intended to be just that. It has been designed and written so that the diagrams and text complement each other, and both are to be consulted. The emphasis has been on the diagrams, and words have been kept to a minimum.

The book has been produced to provide as comprehensive an overview of the subject as any medical or science undergraduate student will need in order to pass and pass well an examination in basic endocrinology. In addition, it is hoped that *Endocrinology at a Glance* will be useful to students of clinical endocrinology who need to refer rapidly to the mechanisms underlying the subject. The book is not presented as an alternative to the several excellent textbooks of endocrinology, which serve as useful reference texts, and some of which have been used during the writing of this book.

Every attempt has been made to present the data accurately and to provide the most up-to-date and reliable information available. When speculative data are given, their fragility has been indicated. Nevertheless, every writer, especially this one, is human, and if the reader spots errors or a lack of clarity, or has any suggestions to improve or add to the presentation, this feedback will be gratefully appreciated and acknowledged.

I should like to thank the many undergraduate medical, dental and science students who have scrutinized and used the diagrams, or similar ones, over the years, and whose criticisms have helped to make them more useful. I should also like to thank Elizabeth Bridges, Kay Chan, Yacoub Dhaher, Munther Khamashta and Adam Greenstein for reading and commenting on some of the work. It has been a pleasure working with the staff of Blackwell Science Ltd, and particularly Dr Stuart Taylor and Emma Lynch, whose friendly encouragement and advice cheered me on.

Ben Greenstein
London 1994

1 Endocrine glands

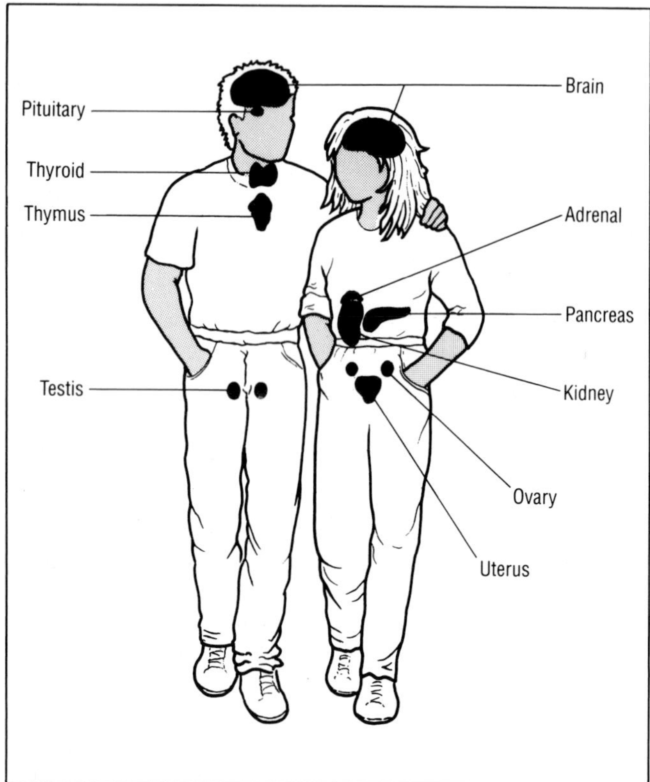

Fig. 1.1 Endocrine glands.

Many aspects of body function are controlled by the endocrine and nervous systems. Both maintain the internal environment in a state of homeostasis, and enable it to alter in response to changes in the external environment. The endocrine system does this by means of *glands* which secrete chemicals or *hormones*. The term *endocrine* refers to a gland that releases the chemicals directly into the extracellular compartment and thence into the bloodstream.

THE PRINCIPAL ENDOCRINE GLANDS

The brain is the controller of the nervous system, but it is also one of the most important endocrine glands. Specialized nerve cells in certain parts of the brain, notably the hypothalamus, synthesize hormones which are transported along the axon to the nerve terminal. Here they are released into the portal blood system, which carries them to the pituitary gland, just beneath the hypothalamus. In some cases, the axon of the neuroendocrine cell projects down to the pituitary cell itself (see page 23). These hormones control, for example, salt and water balance, sexual function and behaviour, lactation and the body's response to stress.

The principal neurohormones known to be synthesized by the brain are:

1 corticotrophin-releasing hormone (CRF; CRH);
2 dopamine (prolactin-inhibiting hormone; PIF);
3 growth-hormone-releasing hormone (GRH; somatocrinin);
4 gonadotrophin-releasing hormone (GnRH; LHRH);
5 somatostatin (growth-hormone-inhibiting hormone; GHIH);
6 thyrotrophin-releasing hormone (TRH);
7 oxytocin;
8 vasopressin.

The pituitary gland synthesizes several hormones which control the function of many of the other endocrine glands. These hormones are synthesized in different cell types of different lobes of the pituitary. The pituitary gland is composed, anatomically, of two lobes, anterior and posterior, which arise from different embryological origins. The anterior pituitary grows upwards, as an outpouching of ectoderm from the floor of the embryonic oral cavity. The posterior pituitary grows down from the base of the brain and therefore has a neural origin. The two lobes become closely apposed to each other to form the pituitary gland. Humans have a miniscule *intermediate lobe*, which is much larger in some other animals.

The principal hormones of the pituitary gland are as follows.

1 *Anterior*:
(a) corticotrophin (adrenocorticotrophic hormone; ACTH);
(b) follicle-stimulating hormone (FSH);
(c) luteinizing hormone (LH);
(d) prolactin (PRL);
(e) thyrotrophin (thyroid-stimulating hormone; TSH);
(f) growth hormone (somatotrophin; GH).

2 *Posterior*:
(g) oxytocin;
(h) vasopressin.

3 *Intermediate lobe*:
(i) melanocyte-stimulating hormone (MSH).

The thyroid gland. In humans, the thyroid gland adheres to, and is situated just in front of the trachea (and behind the larynx). The thyroid-hormone-producing cells, which are arranged in groups or follicles, have a powerful mechanism for concentrating iodine which is used for the synthesis of the thyroid hormone. The circulating hormones are *thyroxine* (T_4) and *tri-iodothyronine* (T_3). In the target tissues, T_3 is the active metabolite of T_4.

The parathyroid glands, which are embedded in the thyroid, produce *parathyroid hormone (parathormone; PTH)*.

PTH plays an important part in the control of levels of calcium and phosphate in the blood.

The parafollicular cells are also in the thyroid, scattered between the thyroid follicles. They produce *calcitonin*.

The adrenal glands are situated just above the kidneys, and are composed of an outer layer, or cortex, and an inner layer, or medulla. The two layers have different functions: the cortex produces steroid hormones and the medulla produces the catecholamines. The adrenal medulla is a modified ganglion. The hormones produced are:

1 *cortex*

(a) the glucocorticoids, principally cortisol in humans, are involved in the control of carbohydrate metabolism

(b) the mineralocorticoids, principally aldosterone, control electrolyte balance

2 *medulla*

(c) adrenaline (called epinephrine in the USA);

(d) noradrenaline (norepinephrine).

[In chemical terms, the prefix nor- denotes the removal of a methyl (CH_3) group from a molecule.]

The endocrine pancreas consists of islet cells scattered in the larger exocrine pancreas, which lies adjacent to the stomach. (The term 'exocrine' refers to glands which have ducts, and which are not covered in this book.) The endocrine pancreas contains cells which secrete the hormones:

1 insulin;
2 glucagon;
3 somatostatin;
4 pancreatic polypeptide.

The ovary is the major female reproductive gland, and produces:

1 oestrogens;
2 progesterone;
3 relaxin.

The testis is the major male reproductive gland, and produces:

1 testosterone;
2 inhibin;
3 Müllerian regression (or inhibiting) factor (fetus).

The ovaries and testes are termed the *gonads*.

The gastrointestinal tract (GIT) is the largest endocrine organ and produces several autocrine, paracrine and endocrine hormones:

1 cholecystokinin (CCK);
2 gastric inhibitory peptide (GIP);
3 gastrin;
4 neurotensin;
5 secretin;
6 substance P;
7 vasoactive intestinal peptide (VIP).

Many of these are also synthesized in the brain, although their role there is far from clear and there may be further hormones as yet undiscovered.

The pineal gland is situated in the brain and is involved with rhythms, for example, the reproductive rhythms of animals which breed seasonally. Its role in humans is not known for certain. The pineal gland produces *melatonin*.

The kidney is an excretory organ, filtering soluble waste products and drugs from the circulation. It also produces hormones involved in the control of blood pressure and in erythropoiesis (production of red blood cells):

1 renin;
2 erythropoietin.

The placenta, which is the organ of pregnancy serving the developing fetus, produces a great number of hormones, many of which are produced by other glands. Two hormones which are produced primarily by the placenta are:

1 chorionic gonadotrophin (CG; hCG; h, human);
2 placental lactogen (PL).

The thymus, which overlies the heart, is essential for normal fetal growth. The thymus retains immature lymphocytes and processes them to a mature state, thereby playing an important role in the immune system. The organ produces and secretes several peptides into the circulation, and it is becoming apparent that these may be important hormones. They include:

1 the thymosin family of peptides;
2 thymopoietin;
3 thymulin.

A number of other hormones and growth factors are produced by the organs, for example, vitamin D by the liver, skin and kidneys.

2 Chemical transmission

Hormones are chemical messengers which are present in the simplest forms of life. Insulin has been measured in *Escherichia coli*, a bacterium, proving that hormones evolved very early in the history of living cells. They may be classified several ways, including, for example, in terms of the cells they target.

1 *Autocrine*: acting on the cells which synthesized them. An example is the insulin-like growth factor (IGF-1), which stimulates cell division in the tumour cell which produced it.

2 *Paracrine*: acting on neighbouring or distant cells, separated from each other only by the extracellular space. An example is insulin, which is secreted by B cells in the pancreas and which affects the secretion of another hormone, glucagon, by the A cells, also in the pancreas.

3 *Endocrine*: acting on cells or organs at distant sites, to which they are carried in the bloodstream, or through another aqueous ducting system, such as the lymph. Examples of endocrine hormones are insulin and the sex hormones.

4 *Neuroendocrine*: this is really paracrine or endocrine, except that the hormones are synthesized in a nerve cell (neurone) which releases the hormone adjacent to the target cell (paracrine), or releases it into the bloodstream, which carries it to the target cell. An example of the former is oxytocin, which is transported along the nerve axon to the posterior pituitary gland (see page 68). An example of the latter is the hormone gonadotrophin-releasing hormone (GnRH), which is synthesized in the brain and released into the portal blood system, which carries it to cells in the anterior pituitary gland (see page 66).

5 *Neural*: this is neurotransmission, which is a form of paracrine effect, when a chemical is released by one neurone and acts on an adjacent neurone, usually to excite or inhibit its electrical and/or chemical activity. These chemicals are termed *neurotransmitters*, for example, acetylcholine and noradrenaline. Neurotransmitters produce virtually instantaneous effects, whereas some chemicals have a slower onset but longer lasting effect on the target organ, and are termed *neuromodulators*. Some of the endogenous, morphine-like peptides, such as the endorphins (see page 35), are neuromodulators.

6 *Pheromonal* transmission is the release of volatile hormones, called pheromones, into the atmosphere, where they are transmitted to another individual, usually of the same species, and are recognized as an olfactory signal. Some have been identified, for example, civetone secreted by the civet, and bombykol, secreted by the silkworm moth.

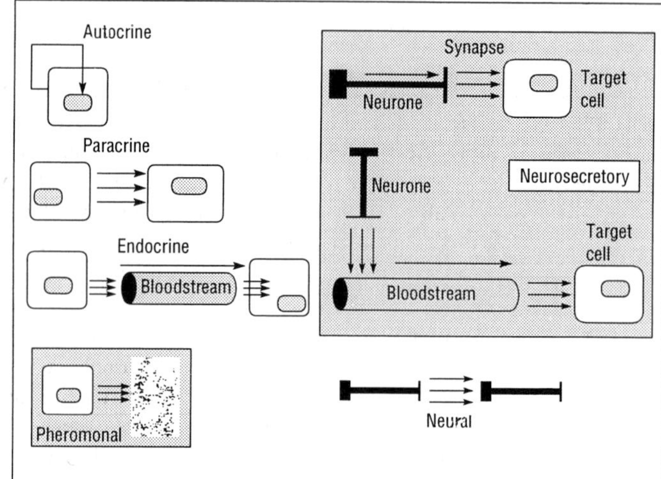

Fig. 2.1 Chemical transmission.

BASIC PRINCIPLES OF NEUROTRANSMISSION

Neurotransmission is becoming increasingly important in the study of endocrinology as the role of the brain as an endocrine gland becomes clearer. It is therefore essential to outline some of the basic principles which will be referred to later in the book.

When the nerve impulse arrives at the terminal, it triggers a calcium-dependent fusion of neurotransmitter packets or vesicles with the nerve terminal plasma membrane, followed by release of the neurotransmitter into the gap, or synapse, between the nerve cells. The neurotransmitters and neuromodulators bind to specific plasma membrane receptors, which transmit the information that the neurotransmitter has bound by means of other membrane proteins and intracellular 'second messengers'. The cell responds appropriately.

The neurotransmitters dissociate from the receptor and are inactivated by enzymes (e.g. in the case of acetylcholine), or taken up into the nerve that released them and metabolized (e.g. noradrenaline). The release of the neurotransmitter may be modulated and limited by (i) autoreceptors on the nerve terminal from which it was released, so that further release of the neurotransmitter is inhibited; and (ii) by presynaptic inhibition, when another neurone synapses with the nerve terminal.

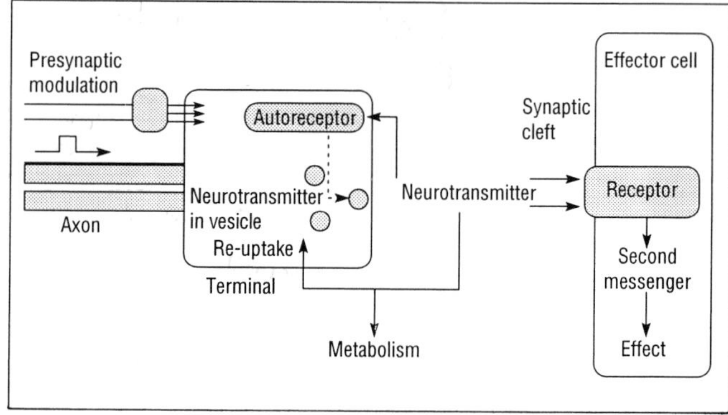

Fig. 2.2 Nerve terminal.

CHEMICAL TRANSPORT

The movement of chemicals between cells and organs is in many cases tightly controlled in order to maintain adequate concentrations in the appropriate compartments of tissues that synthesize, use, transport and metabolize them. Several mechanisms are involved, depending on the nature of the chemical and the environment in which the chemical moves.

Diffusion is the movement of molecules in a fluid phase, and in random thermal (sometimes called Brownian) motion. If two solutions containing the same chemical, one concentrated and the other relatively dilute, are separated by a membrane which is completely permeable and passive, the concentrations of the chemical on either side of the membrane will eventually end up being the same. This is because there are many molecules of the chemical on the concentrated side, and therefore a statistically greater probability of movement from the more concentrated side to the more dilute side of the membrane. Eventually, when the concentrations are equal on both sides, the net change on either side becomes zero. Lipophilic (fat-soluble) molecules such as ethyl alcohol and the steroids diffuse freely across all biological membranes.

Facilitated transport (also called facilitated diffusion) is the transport of chemicals across membranes by carrier proteins which do not need energy to do so. Therefore, they cannot transport chemicals against a concentration gradient. The mechanism can be specific, in that other substances with similar structures to the carried molecule will compete for transport by the carrier proteins. The numbers of transporter proteins may be under hormonal control. Glucose, for example, is carried into the cell by transporter proteins whose numbers are increased by insulin (see page 78).

Active transport is similar to facilitated transport, in that chemicals are helped across the membrane by proteins within it. In addition, the process uses energy in the form of adenosine triphosphate (ATP) or other metabolic fuels. Therefore, chemicals can be transported across the membrane against a concentration gradient, and the transport process can be interrupted by metabolic poisons or other causes of a lack of energy.

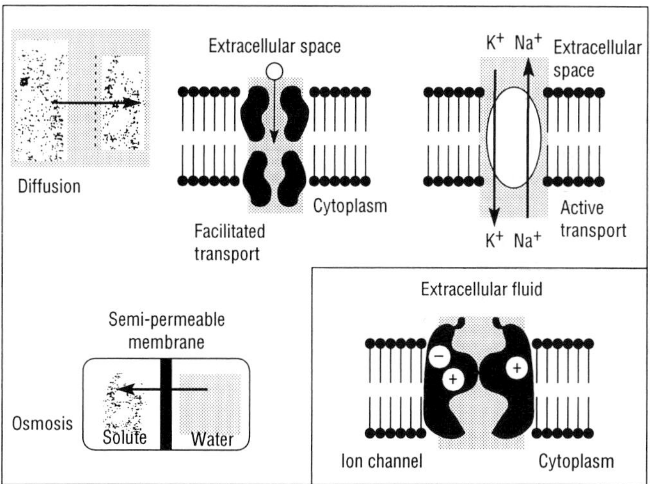

Fig. 2.3 Chemical transport.

Active transport is similar to an enzyme-catalysed reaction in some respects: it is subject to steady-state kinetics. When efflux = influx, no net movement of chemicals occurs. An enzyme binds a substrate with high affinity, and uses energy to convert it into a product which it releases easily. An active transport protein binds the molecule to be transported with high affinity on one side of the membrane, and uses energy to transport it to the other side, where it releases the molecule unchanged. Ions such as Na^+ and K^+ are moved across membranes by active transport.

Ion channels mediate active transport, and consist of proteins containing charged amino acids that may form activation and inactivation 'gates'. Ion channels may be activated by receptors, or by voltage changes through the cell membrane. Channels of the ion Ca^{2+} can be activated by these two methods.

Osmosis is the passive movement of water through a semipermeable membrane, from a compartment of low solute concentration to one which has a greater concentration of the solute. ('Solute' refers to the chemical which is dissolved in the 'solvent', usually water, in biological tissues.) Cells will shrink or swell depending on the concentrations of the solutes on either side of the membrane.

Phagocytosis and pinocytosis are both examples of endocytosis, which is the method whereby substances can enter the cell without having to pass through the cell membrane. Phagocytosis is the ingestion or 'swallowing' of a solid particle by a cell, while pinocytosis is the ingestion of fluid. Receptor-mediated endocytosis is the ingestion of specifically recognized substances by coated pits. These are parts of the membrane which are coated with specific membrane proteins, which include a protein called *clathrin*.

Exocytosis is the movement of substances out of the cell. Neurotransmitters and hormones which are stored in the small vesicles or packets are secreted or released from the cell in which they are stored by exocytosis, when the vesicle fuses with the membrane.

Hormone transport in blood is a very important part of endocrine function. When hormones are secreted into the blood, many are immediately bound to plasma proteins. The proteins may recognize the hormone specifically, and bind it with high affinity and specificity, for example, the binding of sex hormones by SHBG (see page 51). Other proteins, such as albumin, also bind many hormones, including thyroid hormone and the sex hormones, with much lower affinity (i.e. not so tightly).

An equilibrium is set up between the free and bound hormone, so that a fixed proportion of the hormone travels free and unbound, while most is carried bound. It is currently believed that only the free fraction of the hormone is physiologically active and available to the tissues and for metabolism. When a hormone is bound to plasma proteins, it is physiologically inactive and is also protected from metabolic enzymes in organs such as the liver. Plasma binding of hormones is also important in drug interactions, since some drugs, such as aspirin, can displace other substances from their binding sites on the albumin molecule.

3 Mechanisms of hormone action: I

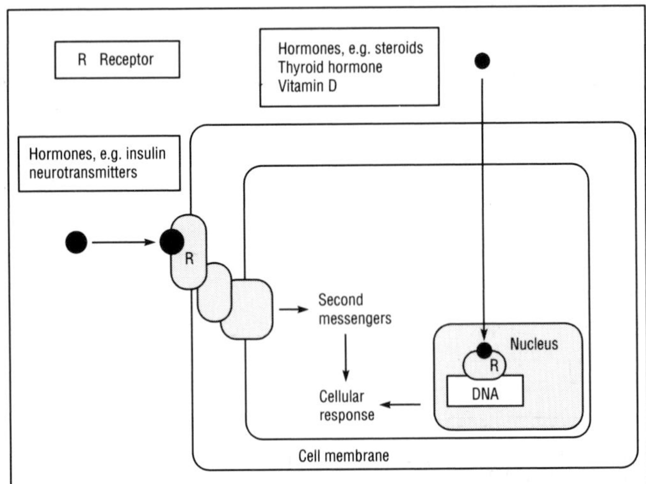

Fig. 3.1 Mechanisms of hormone action.

Hormones interact with their target cells through a primary interaction with receptor proteins which recognize the hormones selectively, thus conferring specificity of response. Charged molecules such as peptides and neurotransmitters bind to receptors on the cell membrane. This causes a conformational change in other membrane proteins, which activate enzymes inside the cell, resulting in the synthesis of 'second messengers', which activate phosphorylating enzymes.

Uncharged molecules, such as the steroid hormones, thyroid hormone and vitamin D, diffuse into the cell and bind to receptor proteins which may be in the cytoplasm or nucleus. The hormone–receptor complex binds to specific hormone response elements (HRE) on the DNA, and mRNA and protein synthesis are altered as a result. This means that the cell will react faster to peptides and neurotransmitters than it will to hormones, which work through relatively slow changes in protein synthesis.

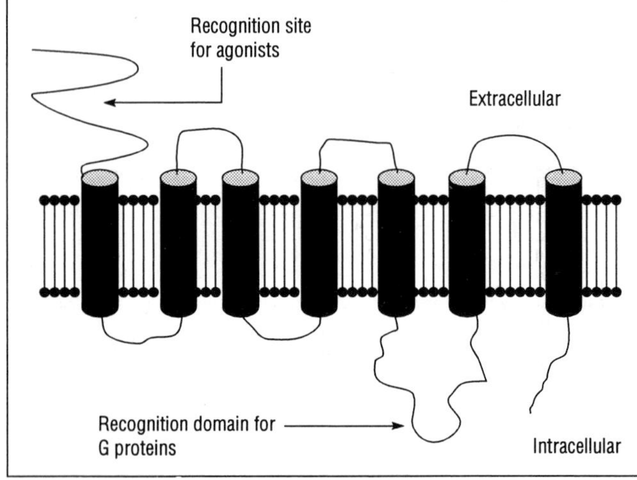

Fig. 3.3 Membrane receptor structure.

MEMBRANE RECEPTORS

Three regions can be distinguished in membrane receptors: the extracellular; the membrane-spanning; and the intracellular domains. The extracellular, N-terminal domain has the hormone-binding domain, and also has glycosylation sites, although it is not known whether these carbohydrate additions to the molecule play any part in hormone binding. The extracellular domain which binds the receptor is often rich in cysteine residues, which form rigid pockets in which the hormone is bound. The transmembrane region consists of one or more segments, made up of hydrophobic (uncharged) amino acids, arranged helically, whose role may include the anchoring of the receptor in the membrane. Different subunits within the membrane may be held together by means of S–S linkages (e.g. the insulin receptor, page 78). The intracellular domain is the effector region of the receptor, which may be linked with another membrane protein system, a set of enzymes which are guanosine triphosphatases (GTPases). The beta-adrenergic receptor is an example of a G-protein-linked receptor. Another class, which includes the insulin receptor, has the intracellular domain as a tyrosine protein kinase. The intracellular region may also have a regulatory tyrosine or serine/threonine phosphorylation site.

SECOND MESSENGERS

The hormone binds to the receptor, which activates a membrane G protein, which moves to the receptor. In the inactive state, the G protein binds GDP, which is exchanged for GTP, and a subunit of the G protein activates adenylate cyclase to convert ATP to the second messenger cyclic AMP. Adenylate cyclase is situated on the plasma membrane, but does not itself bind the hormone. Once formed in the cytoplasm, cAMP activates the catalytic subunit of a specific protein kinase (PKA), which forms part of a cascade of intracellular phosphorylations resulting in the cellular response. Since just one molecule of hormone can result in the production of many molecules of cAMP, this is a very efficient means of amplifying the receptor–hormone interaction. Once formed, cAMP is rapidly broken down by the enzyme phosphodiesterase. An example of a hormone operating through adenylate cyclase is *adrenaline*, through the adrenergic beta receptor.

Hormones can produce inhibitory effects on a cell, and this may be achieved through the fact that some G proteins, such as G_I, may inhibit adenylate cyclase, thus inhibiting the formation of cAMP. An example of this mechanism in action is the inhibition of adenylate cyclase through the binding of *noradrenaline* to the alpha-2-receptor on the presynaptic nerve terminal.

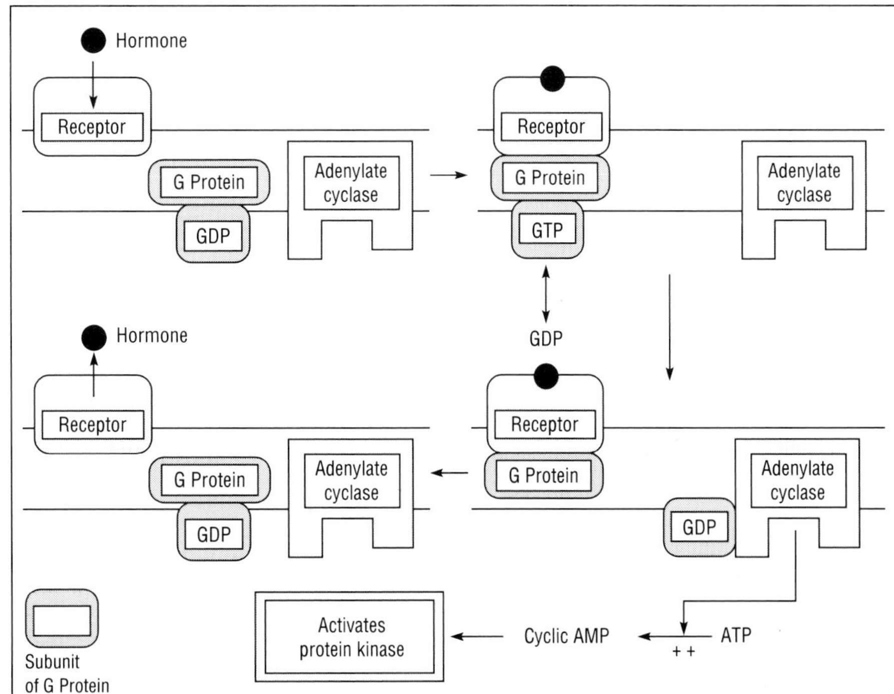

Fig. 3.3 cAMP as second messenger.

INOSITOL TRIPHOSPHATE SYSTEM

In this system, the hormone–receptor–G-protein complex interaction triggers the membrane enzyme phospholipase C (PLC), which catalyses the hydrolysis of phosphoinositol (PIP_2) to two important metabolites, inositol triphosphate (IP_3) and diacylglycerol (DAG). IP_3 generates from the endoplasmic endothelium, increased free Ca^{2+}, which together with DAG promotes the activation and migration to the membrane of the enzyme protein kinase C (PKC). PKC may also be mobilized through the entry of Ca^{2+} into the cell. Examples of hormones and neurotransmitters which activate the system are *adrenaline* acting on alpha-1 receptors and *acetylcholine* on muscarinic cholinergic receptors.

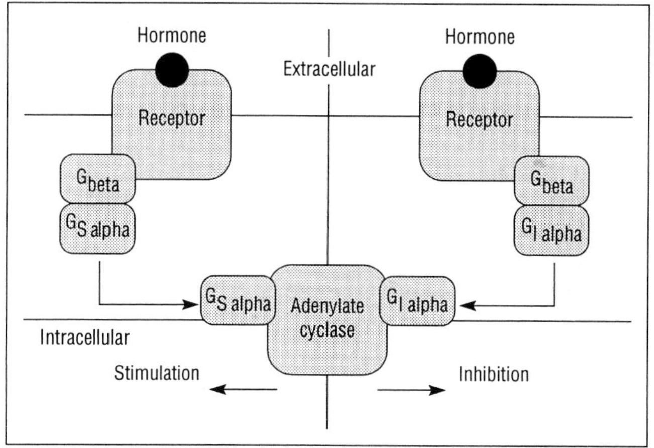

Fig. 3.4 Adenyl cyclase.

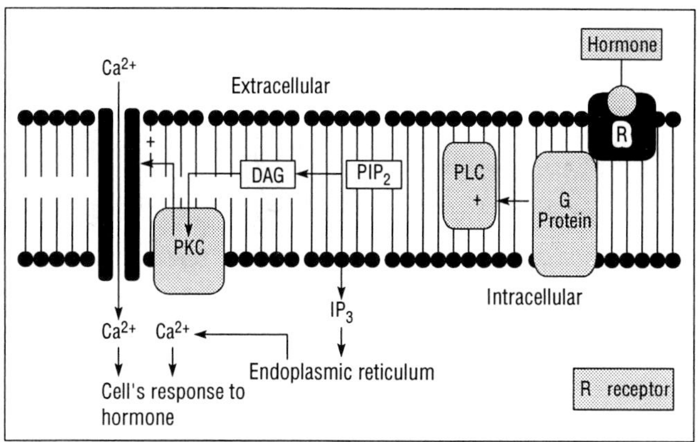

Fig. 3.5 Inositol triphosphate system.

4 Mechanisms of hormone action: II

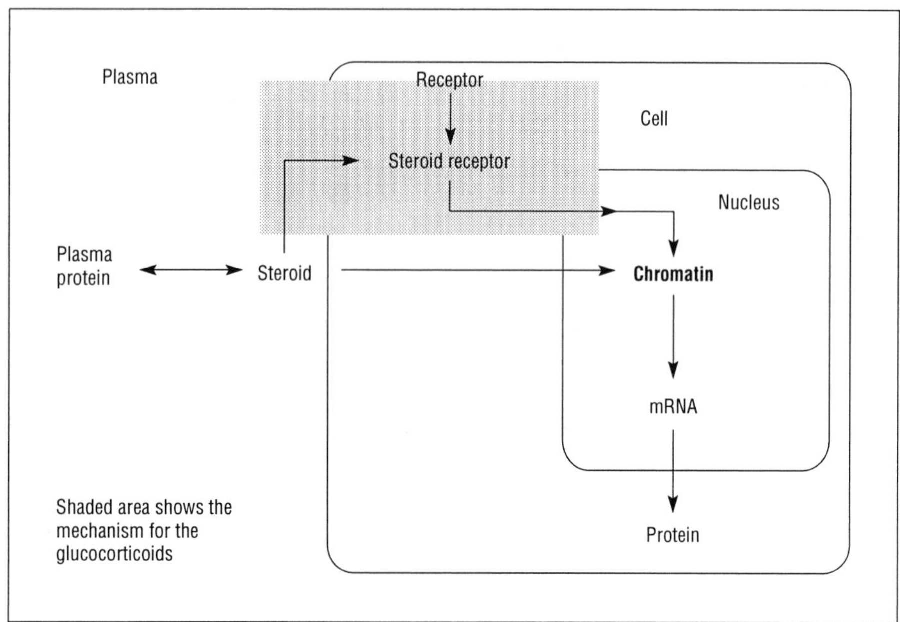

Fig. 4.1 Intracellular receptors.

INTRACELLULAR RECEPTORS

Lipophilic hormones such as the steroids, glucocorticoids and the sex hormones, thyroid hormone and vitamin D, pass easily through the plasma membrane into the cell, where they combine with specific receptor proteins. All the examples mentioned here act via their receptors to alter transcription. In the case of the thyroid hormone and the sex hormones, the receptor is in the nucleus, while in the case of the glucocorticoids, the receptor is in the cytoplasm, and after the hormone binds to it, the complex is translocated to the nucleus.

In the inactive state, for the subfamily of glucocorticoid, progesterone, oestrogen and androgen receptors, the receptor is bound to a protein, a heat shock protein (HSP90). The 90 refers to the size of the protein. The proteins are so called because they were discovered in heat-traumatized cells. The proteins are associated with disease, fever, ischaemia, ageing and the inflammatory process, but their functions are unclear.

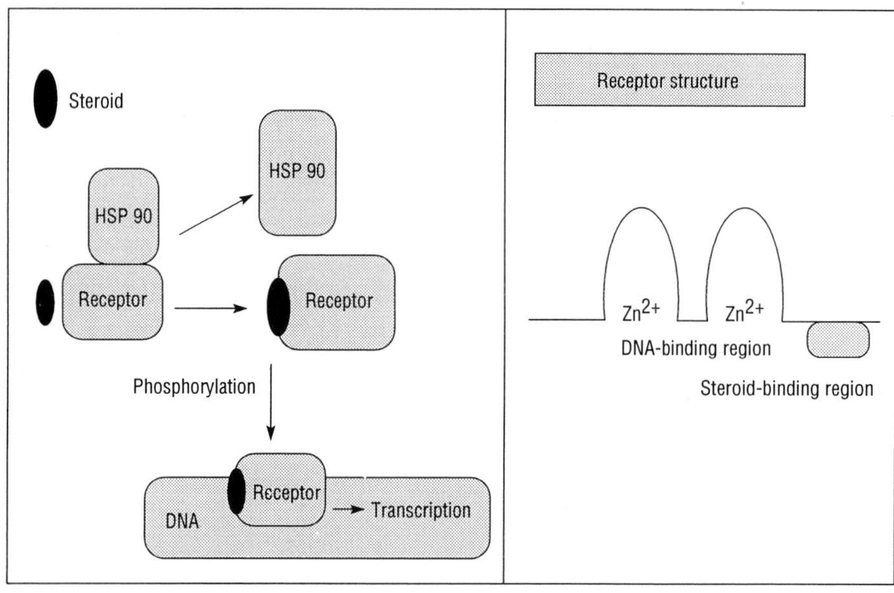

Fig. 4.2 Heat shock proteins and zinc fingers.

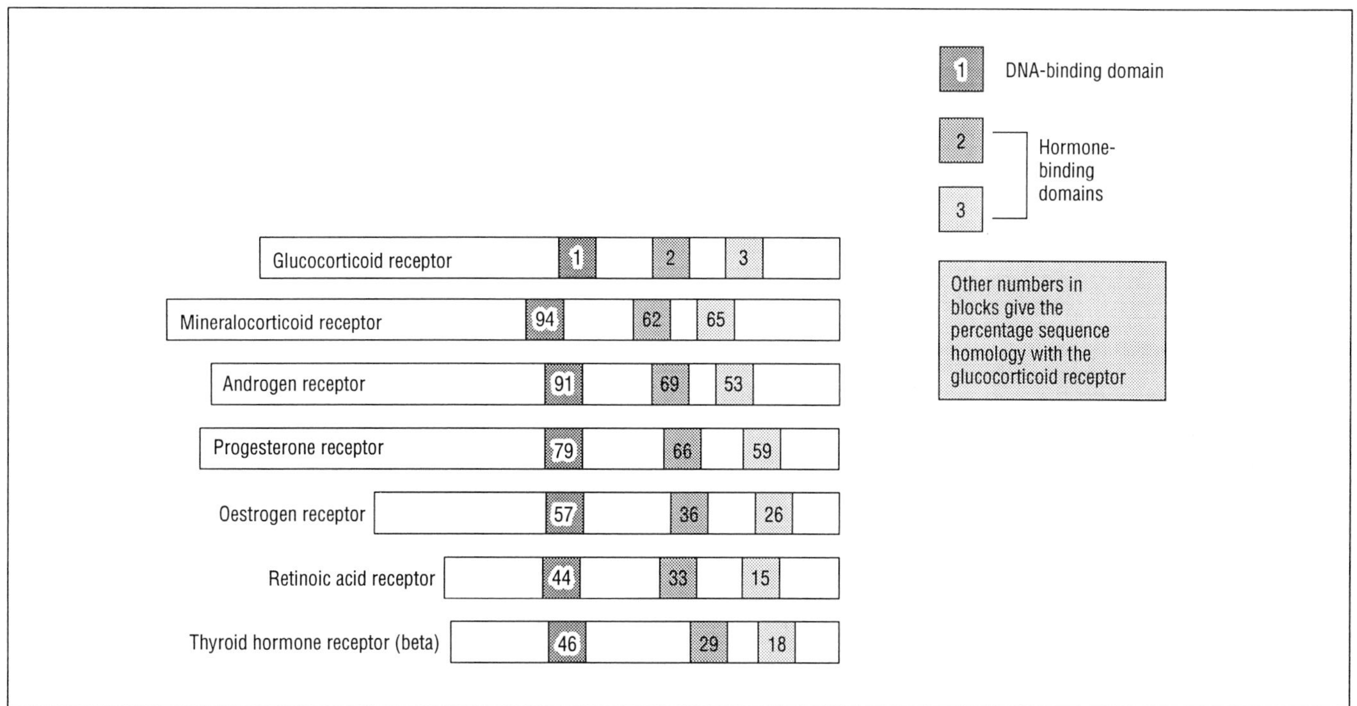

Fig. 4.3 Members of steroid receptor superfamily.

When the hormone binds to the receptor, the HSP dissociates from it, the receptors form homodimers (two receptor molecules associate) and the hormone–receptor complex binds to the DNA at specific sites, termed hormone response elements (HREs), which lie upstream from transcription initiation sites. Transcription and subsequent protein synthesis are altered. The thyroid hormone and retinoic acid receptors are not associated with HSPs in their inactive state, and are able to associate with their response elements on the DNA in the absence of the hormones. The activation of receptors, so that they can express the actions of the hormones, appears to be achieved through their phosphorylation, although at present this process is poorly understood.

NATURE OF THE STEROID RECEPTOR

The steroid receptors form part of a larger 'superfamily' of nuclear DNA-binding receptors, including thyroid and vitamin D receptors. They all have two main regions, a hydrophobic hormone-binding region and a DNA-binding region, which consists of two 'zinc fingers', rich in cysteine and basic amino acids. The structures of the receptors are known. Region 1 is the DNA-binding region, and is the most conserved among the members of the receptor family, in that it has a high sequence homology from receptor to receptor, as shown in the scheme above. It is thought that the first zinc finger determines the specificity of the binding of the receptor to DNA, while the second finger stabilizes the receptor to its response element of the DNA. Regions 2 and 3 of the receptors determine the hormone specificity of binding, and are not well conserved among the different receptors.

Cloning of steroid receptor cDNA has revealed the existence of 'orphan receptors'. These are proteins which form a very large proportion of the steroid receptor superfamily, but for which no natural ligand or function has yet been found.

5 Hormone antagonism

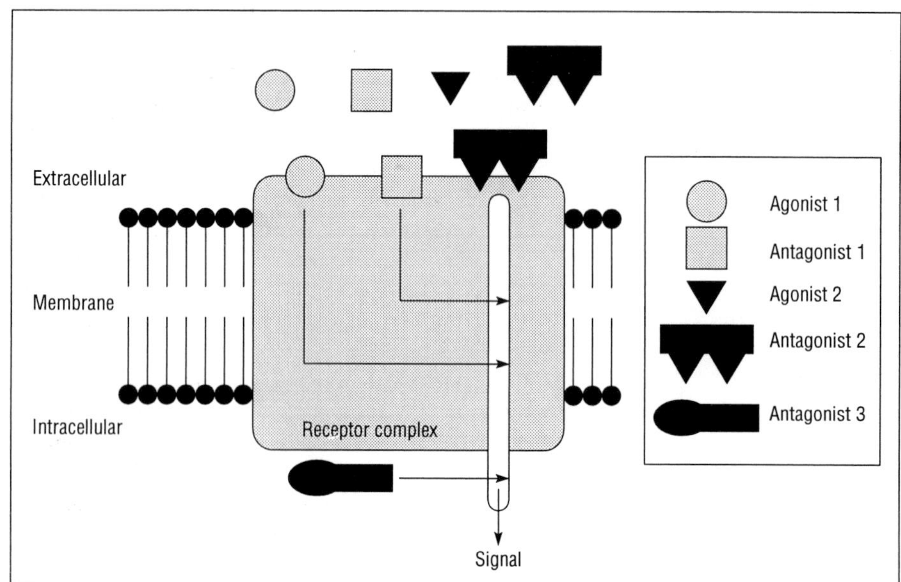

Fig. 5.1 Hormone antagonism.

RECEPTOR ANTAGONISM

Antagonism of hormone–receptor interactions is a very important aspect of endocrinology, not only in terms of the study of the hormone–receptor interaction, but also in therapeutic terms, since antagonists play a large part in the treatment of endocrine-based disease. Antagonists can block the actions of the hormone in a number of ways. The examples shown illustrate some of the known mechanisms of antagonist action on receptors located on the surface of the cell. The stylized receptor is presented with several different targets for antagonist action, although in nature one receptor may not possess all these targets for antagonist attack. In classical pharmacological terms, the molecule or ligand which binds to the receptor and elicits the normal cellular response is termed the *agonist*. The ligand which binds but which elicits no response is the *antagonist*.

In the case shown, two molecules of agonist 2 are required to bind to their receptor sites in order to initiate a response.

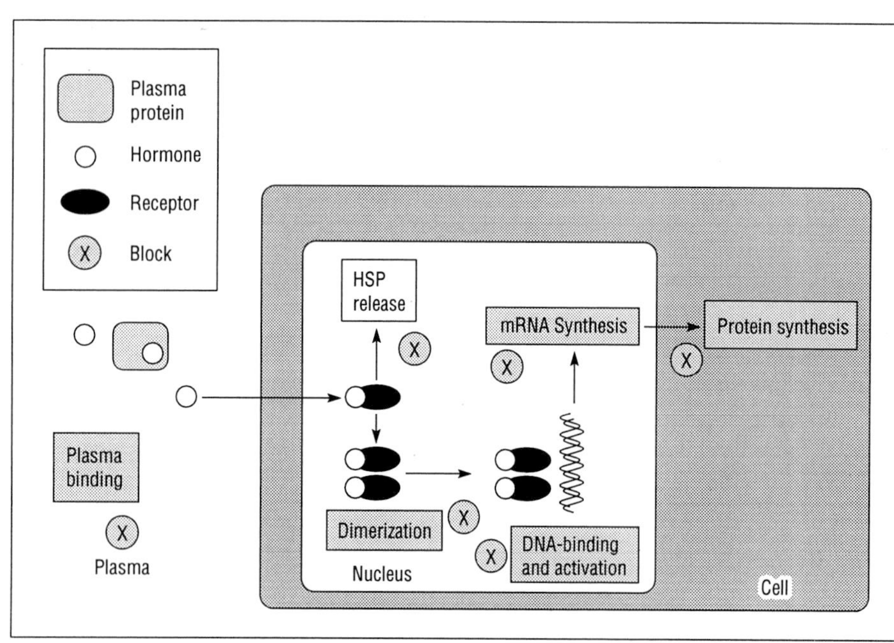

Fig. 5.2 Sites of intracellular hormone antagonism.

Antagonist 2 binds to both sites and prevents the hormone from gaining access. A good example of this is the neurotransmitter *acetylcholine*: two molecules bind to their receptor sites and the binding is inhibited by the antagonist tubocurarine. In another case, agonist 1 binds to its site in order to elicit the cellular response, whereas antagonist 1 binds to another, allosteric site in order to block the response. A possible example is the neurotransmitter *glutamate*, which binds to its receptor in order to open ion channels, and the antagonist 2, aminophosphonovalerate, may bind to an allosteric site to block glutamate action. Antagonist 3 is able to penetrate the membrane, or pass completely through it into the cell, where it blocks the signal after it has been generated by the normal agonist–receptor interaction. An example of antagonist 3 is the anticonvulsant drug phenytoin, which physically blocks the ion channel.

Hormone augmentation. Note that although it is principally hormone antagonism which is being described here, hormone action can be potentiated through the receptors, or at post-receptor sites. For example, the action of glutamate on its receptor is potentiated by an allosteric binding of another neurotransmitter, *glycine*, to a receptor site on the membrane receptor complex. In another well-known case, the action of adrenaline is potentiated through the action of a group of substances called *xanthines*, for example, *caffeine*, which block the enzyme phosphodiesterase, which breaks down adrenaline's second messenger, cAMP.

INTRACELLULAR RECEPTOR ANTAGONISTS

Hormone action in the cell can be blocked by substances which interfere with the processing of the normal intracellular hormone–receptor interaction. This can occur at one or more of several sites. The receptor itself may be blocked, or the post-receptor events, such as mRNA or protein synthesis, inhibited.

RECEPTOR-BLOCKING ANTAGONISTS

Terminology note: Readers will often come across the term *partial agonist* when studying steroid hormone antagonists. Partial agonists are drugs which not only block the action of the hormone, but under some conditions will actually be able to produce a response similar to that of the natural hormone.

Dimerization block. Antagonists have been developed to the steroid hormones, and particularly to the sex hormones. Their uses will be referred to later on, but they are also mentioned here as examples of specific types of hormone antagonists. An example of a drug which may act to block dimerization of the oestrogen receptor is the synthetic drug *ICI 164384* (ICI is the company that produced it). ICI 164384 appears to inhibit the normal dimerization of the oestrogen receptor by blocking the binding of the sex hormone oestradiol. Failure to dimerize adversely affects the ability of the receptor to bind to the DNA, thus blocking transcription. This is pure antagonism.

Transcriptional block. This is the mechanism whereby two important partial agonists, namely *tamoxifen* and *RU486*, produce their effect. Tamoxifen is an anti-oestrogen, developed by ICI for the treatment of breast cancer, and RU486 is an antiprogestational agent, developed by Roussel, and is used to terminate pregnancy. It has been proposed that there are two transcriptional activation sites on the DNA for the oestrogen and progesterone receptors, called TAF-1 and TAF-2, both functioning independently of each other. There is evidence that the antagonists block TAF-2 selectively, while allowing TAF-1 to operate normally. Therefore, in situations where TAF-2 predominates, tamoxifen and RU486 will act as antagonists; when TAF-1 and TAF-2 are activated, then the drugs will act as mixed antagonists and agonists, that is, as partial agonists.

Non-specific RNA and protein synthesis inhibitors. There are drugs, particularly the antibiotics and antineoplastic (anticancer) drugs, which will block RNA and protein synthesis non-selectively. The toadstool toxin, alpha-amanitin, extracted from the fungus *Amanita phylloides*, selectively blocks mRNA by inhibiting the enzyme RNA polymerase B, while the antibiotic actinomycin D actually intercalates into the DNA to block transcription. The antibiotic tetracyclines inhibit protein synthesis by blocking the translation of expressed mRNA.

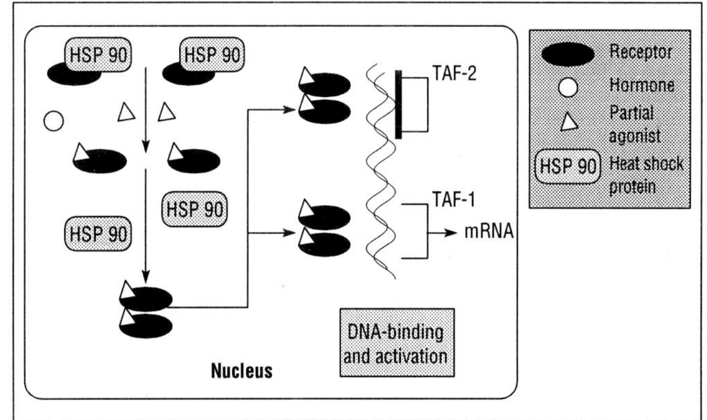

Fig. 5.3 Model of intranuclear partial agonist action.

6 Methods in endocrinology

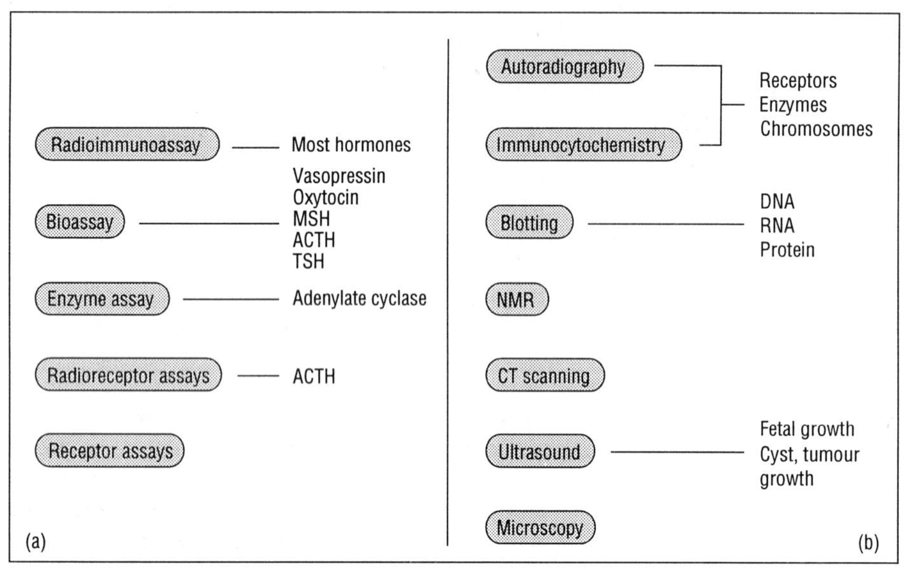

Fig. 6.1 (a) Measurement of hormones, receptors and chemical mediators; (b) detection and visualization.

MEASUREMENT AND LOCALIZATION

Without the ability to measure hormones, receptors and enzyme activity, it would not be possible to study endocrine systems. Hormone secretion alters in response to physiological and pathological conditions, as do receptors and enzyme activity. In addition, we need methods which will enable us to learn the anatomical distribution and state of activity of endocrine mediators.

Hormone measurement. Hormones were first measured by *bioassay*, sometimes even before the hormone had been discovered. For example, extracts of testes were injected into cockerels and their potency determined in terms of comb growth. Pancreatic extracts were injected and the fall in blood glucose measured. Bioassays are still used today, even though hormones have been isolated, since they provide a biological index of hormone activity. Some are sensitive enough to detect physiological concentrations of hormones in blood, for example, the suppressant effect of vasopressin on micturition, the effect of melanocyte-stimulating hormone (MSH) on melanin granules in frog skin, and the effect of adrenocorticotrophic hormone (ACTH) on steroidogenesis in adrenal tissue *in vitro*. Bioassays have several disadvantages. They are not always sensitive enough to detect plasma concentrations of some hormones; they are laborious and sometimes difficult to learn. Often, results may vary between laboratories.

Radioimmunoassay (RIA) was a big advance. RIA was developed after the discovery of antibodies to insulin in the plasma of patients. The antibodies were collected and used to develop the first RIA.

The method relies on the specificity of the antigen–antibody reaction, when an antibody will recognize one antigen (e.g. hormone). The basic method is to mix together a quantity of the antibody to the hormone, and a tracer amount of the radioactively labelled hormone, together with a range of concentrations of unlabelled hormone, which would displace the labelled hormone from its antibody-binding sites. The hormone-bound antibody is separated from unbound hormone, and the radioactivity held by the hormone–antibody complex is measured. From this experiment, a standard curve showing the displacement of bound radioactive hormone by increasing amounts of unlabelled hormone can be prepared. A sample of plasma or other body fluid is mixed with the same amount of antibody and tracer, and the degree of displacement of labelled hormone is checked on the standard curve against the displacement produced by known amounts of hormone.

Attempts to make the assay more specific include the preparation of antibodies which will recognize different parts of the hormone, a technique possible only when measuring peptide or protein hormones. When the hormone is a small molecule, it has to be coupled with a carrier protein, such as albumin, in order to raise an antibody to it. RIA is now the most common assay technique for virtually all hormones, and for many other biochemicals. It is extremely sensitive, easily performed, can accommodate very many samples to be measured in one 'run', and is easy to learn. Disadvantages are interlaboratory variability, due to antibody variation, the fact that bioassay and radioimmunoassay do not always give the same result, and the assumption that labelled and unlabelled hormones will bind to the same extent to the antibody. The same principle of measurement can be applied, but using, instead of an antibody, a preparation of the receptors to the hormone, if these are available, although *radioreceptor* assay is usually not as sensitive as RIA.

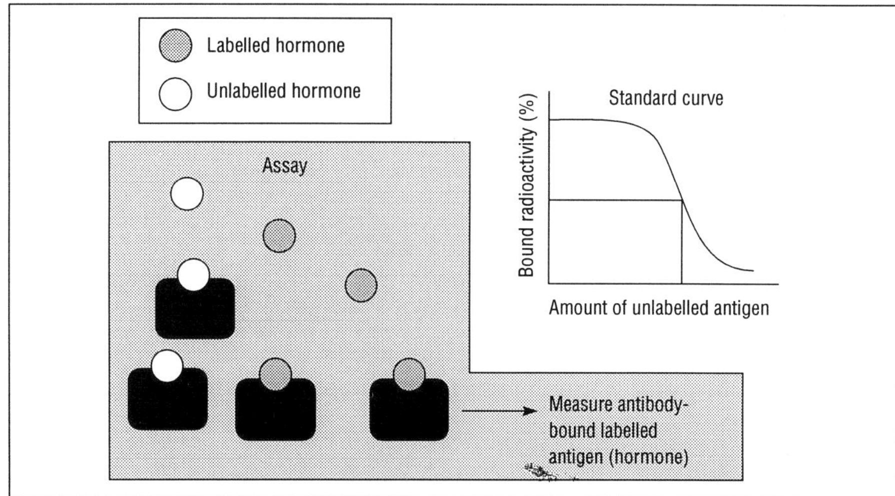

Fig. 6.2 Principles of radioimmunoassay.

Enzyme assay is the measurement of enzyme activity by monitoring changes in substrate conversion to product, for example, the measurement of adenylate cyclase activity through the measurement of the conversion of radiolabelled ATP to cAMP.

Receptor assays are techniques for the measurement of receptor activity, and utilize the same techniques as for RIA. It is assumed that one molecule of radioactive hormone binds to one molecule of the receptor, and using kinetics it is possible to calculate the numbers of receptors in a tissue extract, and also the affinity with which the receptor binds the hormone. This technique is useful in measuring changes in receptor activity, for example, the stimulant effect of oestrogens on progesterone receptors in the uterus and brain during the menstrual cycle (see page 50). It is also a useful screening tool for the discovery of agonists and antagonists for experimental and therapeutic purposes.

DETECTION AND VISUALIZATION

Autoradiography. This method is used to visualize the anatomical or cellular distribution of a radioactive substance in the body after administration *in vivo*; after addition to a medium in which cells are cultured; or after application to a thin section on a slide. In all cases, a thin section has to be made, fixed to a slide, dipped in photographic emulsion and exposed to a sensitive film. The radioactive emissions from the decaying isotope blacken the film and the developed image reflects the distribution of the radioactivity. This method has been used to great effect in determining the distribution of the neurotransmitter and steroid hormone receptors in the brain, and in the examination of the function of enzymes involved in endocrine tissues. The method allows the mapping of genes to chromosomes, after the incorporation of radioactive thymidine into growing cells, and the visualization of newly synthesized RNA, which has been transcribed in the presence of radioactive uridine, a constituent of RNA. The ability to label proteins and nucleic acids also has a use in molecular studies of endocrine function, and *blotting* techniques, in which mRNA, DNA or proteins are newly synthesized, utilizes autoradiography to determine the expression of these cellular products after hormonal or genetic manipulation.

Immunocytochemistry is used for the same basic purpose as autoradiography, namely, to visualize and detect specific substances on a slide. It is rapidly replacing autoradiography, as researchers seek sensitive non-radioactive methods to replace the more hazardous use of radioactive isotopes. The basic principle is to label the molecule of interest on the slide, whether it be receptor, enzyme or gene product, with an antibody to the molecule, and then to watch the antibody undergo a colour reaction on the slide.

Non-invasive techniques of whole body visualization are becoming much more widely used, especially in clinical medicine, in order to observe internal changes due to development or disease.

Nuclear magnetic resonance (*NMR*) is a technique used to image soft tissues and is based on the absorption of specific radio frequencies by atomic nuclei. NMR can be used, for example, to detect cancers, brain abnormalities and vascular disease.

Computerized tomography (*CT*) is another scanning method whereby the patient or subject receives a series of narrow, highly restricted X-ray beams, as the machine is rotated about the part of the body being examined. These beams are projected onto scintillation crystals, which are more sensitive than X-ray film, and computer-analysed X-ray transmission profiles are converted into visible images of body tissues, varying in shade from black, through grey to white. Thus, for example, CT can distinguish white and grey matter in the brain, and is therefore very useful for the detection of brain tumours.

Ultrasound, or ultrasonography as it is termed for visualizing body structures, is the use of extremely high frequency sound waves (more than 30 kHz) to generate pictures of body structures. A controlled beam is passed into the body, and the echoes of the reflected sound are used to construct an electronic image of the structure. It is widely used in pregnancy for visualizing the growing fetus and charting its growth; for the diagnosis of multiple pregnancy; for localizing the placenta and for the detection of abnormalities of the fetus. Ultrasound has also been used to detect other pathological conditions, such as polycystic ovaries.

7 Principles of feedback control: brain, pituitary and target glands

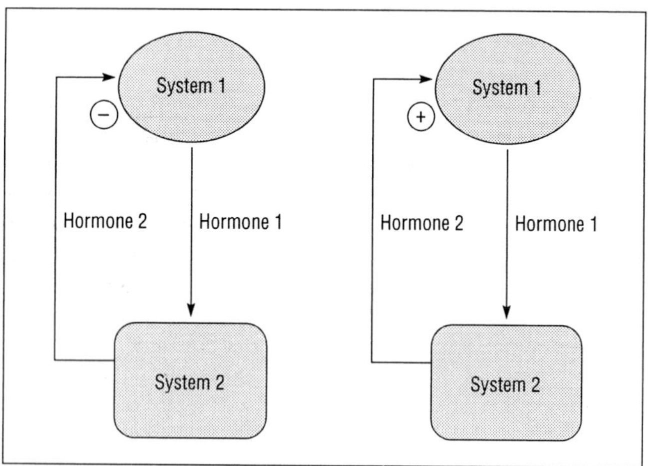

Fig. 7.1 Feedback mechanisms.

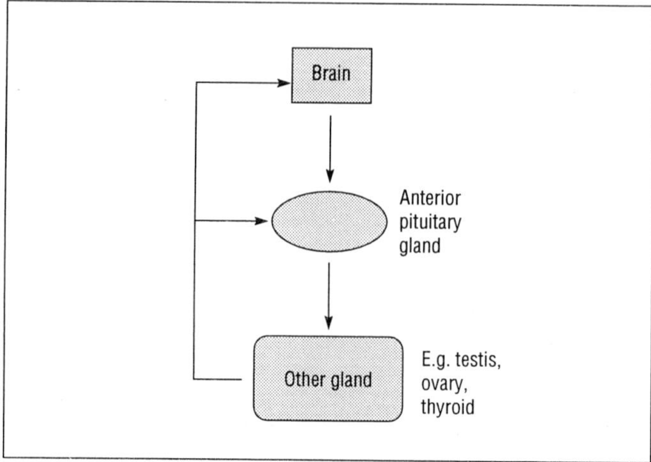

Fig. 7.2 Neuroendocrine axis.

HOMEOSTASIS

Living systems possess their own internal environment, which has to survive within an external environment. Survival involves the maintenance of a fluid and salt balance, a tight control over temperature in the case of homeotherms, and also over the regulation of chemical availability and utilization within the cell. Poikilotherms, whose temperature is set by the external environment, are more dependent on their external environment for maintenance of an adequate metabolism.

Internal control is achieved through the integration of the different systems: neural, biochemical and physical. In all cases, the fundamental components of these systems are: (i) signals; (ii) transducers; (iii) sensors; and (iv) responders. The *signals* may be electrical impulses, or chemicals such as neurotransmitters, hormones, or antigens. The *transducers* are poorly understood coupling systems which transform one form of energy into another, for example, the conversion of an electrical impulse into a quantum of chemical neurotransmitter. *Sensors* are almost always receptor sites in proteins, which recognize

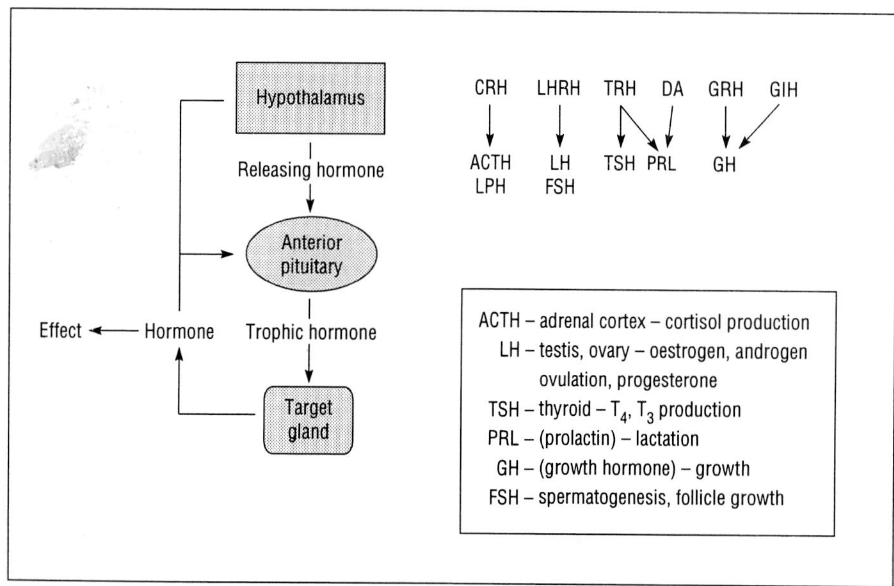

Fig. 7.3 Releasing hormones.

specifically the signals which bind them. Transducers then convert the binding reaction into another electrical or chemical response. *Responders* are the apparatus of the cell that produce the final response, be it release or inhibition of release of a hormone, or of a neurotransmitter.

Integration of the systems is achieved through a complex interplay of regulatory feedback mechanisms operated through the agency of hormonal and neural communication networks. The most important mechanisms are those commonly called *feedback*, whereby systems limit each other's activity around a pre-set oscillator.

For example, system 1 releases a hormone, hormone 1, which causes system 2, another gland, to release another hormone, hormone 2, which travels in the bloodstream. It is sensed by system 1, which compares the concentration of the hormone with a comparator, and responds by altering the output of hormone 1. If system 1 responds by reducing the output of hormone 1, this is called a *negative-feedback* system. An example is the effect of thyroid hormone (hormone 2) from the thyroid gland (system 2), in reducing the output of thyroid-stimulating hormone (TSH; hormone 1) from the anterior pituitary gland (system 1; see page 26).

If system 1 responds by increasing more hormone 1, this is 7
called a *positive-feedback* system. An example is the effect of oestrogen (hormone 2) from the ovary (system 2) on the release of luteinizing hormone (LH; hormone 1) from the anterior pituitary gland (system 1) just before ovulation (see page 49).

In endocrinology, the brain–pituitary–other gland axis provides the most graphic examples of feedback mechanisms in action.

The feedback systems may involve more than two hormones. Take, for example, the control of thyroid hormone secretion. The brain releases a hormone, thyrotrophin-releasing hormone, which travels down the portal blood system (see page 23) to the anterior pituitary thyrotroph cell, where it stimulates the release of TSH. TSH travels in the bloodstream to the thyroid gland, where it stimulates the release of thyroid hormone. Thyroid hormone in turn inhibits TSH release. It will be readily apparent that this sort of system provides a means of testing the proper functioning of the feedback systems in health and disease (see page 27).

8 The neuroendocrine anatomy of the hypothalamus and pituitary gland

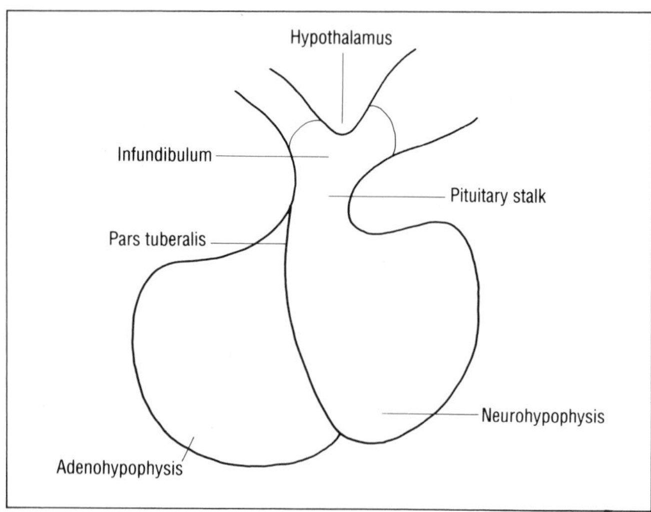

Fig. 8.1 Pituitary gland.

THE HYPOTHALAMUS

The hypothalamus lies at the base of the brain in the diencephalon. It contains a number of groups (or nuclei) of neurones which are important in the regulation of the secretion of hormones from the pituitary. Some of these neurones produce hormones which are transported in the bloodstream to the pituitary and to other parts of the body. The hypothalamus has its boundaries arbitrarily defined in terms of visible structures around it. It has been divided into the rostral or supraoptic hypothalamus; the middle or tuberal hypothalamus; and the caudal or mamillary hypothalamus. Running longitudinally through the middle is the narrow *third ventricle*, which carries the cerebrospinal fluid.

Running from front to back, the hypothalamus is arbitrarily divided into medial and lateral zones. The medial hypothalamus contains a number of nuclei, densely packed with cells, which communicate with the rest of the brain through a bundle of descending and ascending axons: the *medial forebrain bundle*. The lateral zone of the hypothalamus does not have such well-defined nuclei, but has neurones scattered within it.

Looked at from beneath, the hypothalamus lies between: (i) the rostral (nearer the front) *optic chiasm*, where the two optic nerves cross or decussate on their way from the eyes to the visual cortex; and (ii) the caudal (or rear) *mamillary bodies*. In between is a grey swelling, the *tuber cinereum* which tapers to form the *infundibulum*, which is the pituitary stalk. This region is very often termed the *median eminence*. The median eminence is where the vascular link is made between the hypothalamic neurosecretory neurones and the pituitary gland.

The pituitary gland is developmentally and anatomically distinguished as two main sub-glands, namely the anterior and posterior pituitary. (*The pituitary is still referred to as the hypophysis, the anterior gland as the adenohypophysis, and the posterior pituitary gland as the neurohypophysis.*)

Developmentally, the posterior gland is an outgrowth of the brain. During fetal development, it arises as a downward extrusion from the hypothalamus. It is thus neural in origin. The anterior pituitary grows upwards from the primitive oral cavity, which is termed Rathke's pouch. It grows upwards until it fuses with the downgrowing infundibulum, and its cells proliferate around and along the pituitary stalk, giving rise to the *pars tuberalis*. During development, a rich vascular system develops in the median eminence. The upgrowth loses contact with the oral cavity, and the pituitary gland has direct neural contact with the hypothalamus, through to the posterior pituitary, and a vascular link, called the *portal system*, through which chemicals are carried from hypothalamic cells to the anterior pituitary gland.

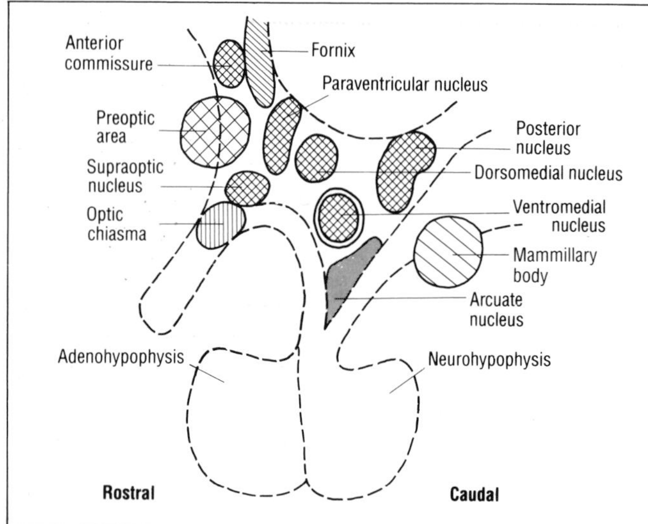

Fig. 8.2 Hypothalamic nuclei.

THE NUCLEI

Supraoptic group of nuclei. The paraventricular (PVN) and supraoptic (SON) nuclei have axons which project to the posterior pituitary as the hypothalamic–hypophyseal tract. The PVN and SON contain large, richly vascularized cells, which together are termed the *magnocellular* secretory system. The PVN has other, smaller cells within it which contribute to a widely diffuse collection of hypothalamic neurones called the *parvocellular* secretory system. The parvocellular system, through the neurohormones it sends to the anterior pituitary, controls anterior pituitary function. Both the SON and PVN contain cells which produce and secrete several important neuropeptides. The PVN is interconnected with autonomic and other regions of the spinal cord and the brain stem, as well as with the pituitary gland.

The suprachiasmatic nuclei, which lie above the optic chiasma, are important in the generation of circadian rhythms of behaviour and hormone secretion.

The tuberal or middle group of nuclei are involved in pituitary regulation. These are the ventromedial, dorsomedial and arcuate nuclei. Like the PVN, the ventromedial is interconnected with other parts of the brain, including the spinal cord, the brain stem and the central grey matter of the mesencephalon (midbrain). The arcuate nucleus, which is an autonomous generator of reproductively important rhythms, sends many axons to the median eminence, as well as to other parts of the hypothalamus and forebrain.

The mammillary or posterior group of nuclei runs caudally into the mesencephalic central grey area and is not as well defined in nuclear organization. Within this area are more magnocellular neurones containing the neurotransmitters gamma-aminobutyric acid (GABA), histamine and the neuropeptide galanin, and these project to many parts of the brain.

THE NEUROHORMONES

The magnocellular neurones of the SON and the PVN contain neurones which produce and secrete *oxytocin* and *vasopressin*. The hormones are produced in different neurones and are transported to the posterior pituitary gland via their axons, which comprise the hypothalamic–hypophyseal tract.

The neurones of the parvocellular neurosecretory system send their axons to the median eminence, where their terminals release the 'releasing hormones': corticotrophin-releasing hormone (CRF); gonadotrophin-releasing hormone (GnRH); thyrotrophin-releasing hormone (TRH); and many other peptides, including somatostatin, also called growth-hormone release-inhibiting factor, and neurotensin. Other substances emptied

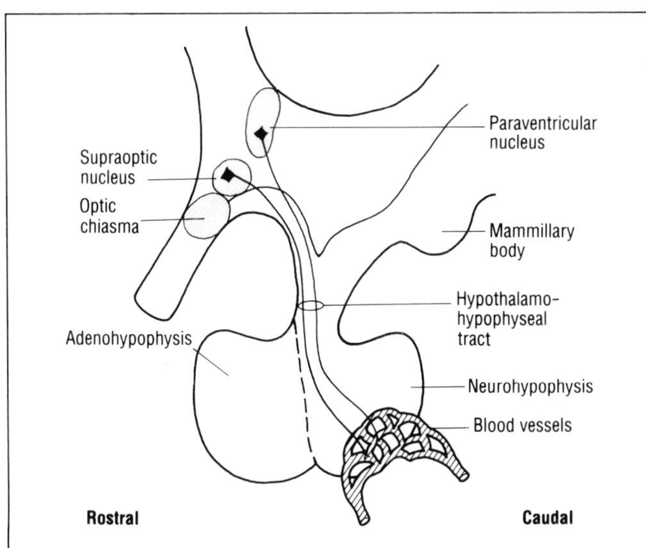

Fig. 8.3 Magnocellular secretory system.

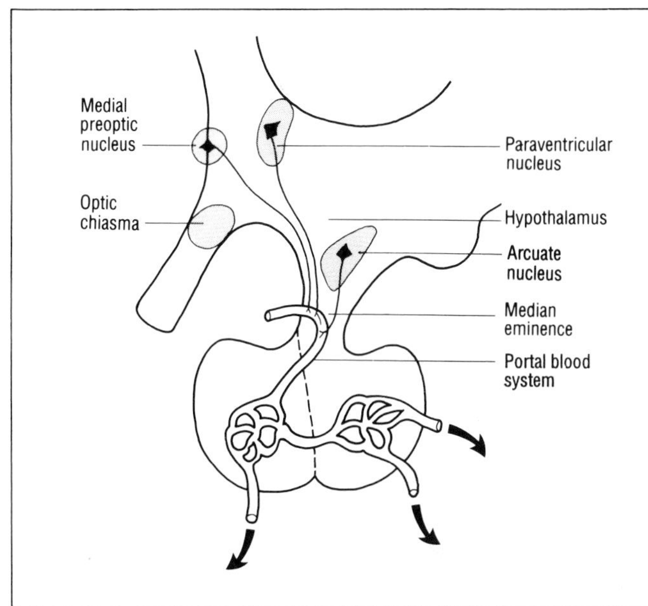

Fig. 8.4 Parvocellular neurosecretory system.

into the portal system include the dynorphins, enkephalins and beta-endorphin, GABA, dopamine, which is also termed prolactin-inhibitory factor in this context, and many more substances.

GnRH neurones have been found mainly in the medial preoptic region and immediately caudal to it. These send axons not only to the median eminence, but to other parts of the brain, giving rise to the idea that GnRH may be a neurotransmitter as well as a prime regulator of fertility.

Cells of the PVN parvocellular system are rich in CRF and TRH, and project to the median eminence. The arcuate nucleus is rich in prolactin neurones, also called tubero-infundibular dopamine neurones. Arcuate neurones also contain the peptides galanin and growth hormone releasing hormone (GRH), the opioids, somatostatin and several other substances, many of which are transported to the median eminence and the portal system.

(*Note: it has been found that in many cases, several neurochemicals may co-exist in one neurone.*)

EXAMPLES OF MAJOR CONNECTING SYSTEMS

The hypothalamus communicates with other parts of itself and with the rest of the brain through several major connecting systems, principally the *medial forebrain bundle (MFB)*, which is rich in noradrenergic neurones, which appear to project principally from the brain stem. The MFB also contains 5HT-containing neurones (serotonergic) which originate in the raphe nuclei of the midbrain. The MFB carries information away from the hypothalamus as well, to the brain stem, spinal cord and to higher centres.

The *stria terminalis* is a major pathway to the medial hypothalamus from the amygdaloid nuclei, an important group of limbic system structures. The *fornix* is the major interconnection between the hippocampus, another limbic structure, and the hypothalamus.

9 The thyroid: I

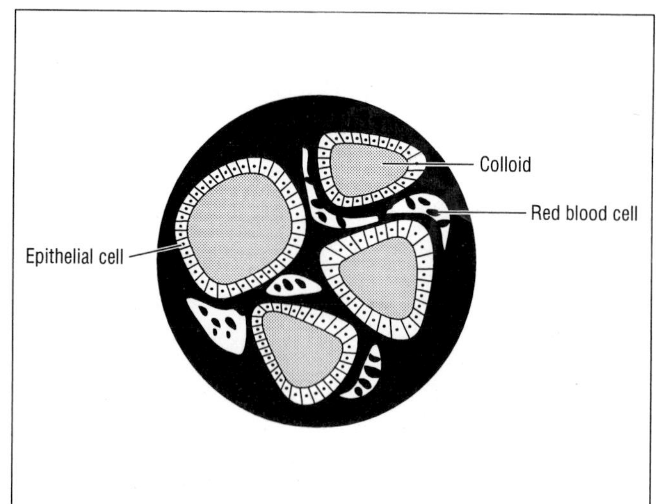

Fig. 9.1 Microscopic appearance of the thyroid gland.

THE GLAND

The human thyroid gland begins to develop at around 4 weeks after conception, and moves down the neck while forming its characteristic bilobular structure, which is completed by the third trimester.

In the normal adult, the gland has two lobes, weighs around 25 g and is situated close to the trachea. The gland is composed of well over a million clusters of cells, or follicles. These are spherical and consist of cells surrounding a central mass or colloid. Each cell has three functions: (i) exocrine, because it secretes substances into the colloid; (ii) absorptive, because it takes up substances from the colloid by pinocytosis (see page 11); endocrine, because it secretes hormones directly in the bloodstream.

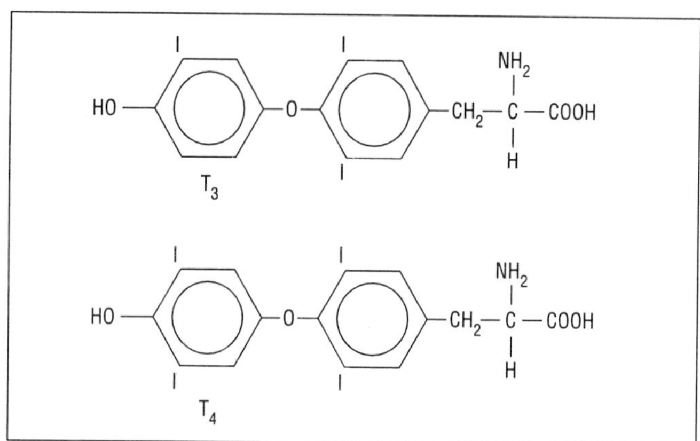

Fig. 9.3 Thyroid hormones.

THE HORMONES

Synthesis. The follicle cells have in their basement membrane an iodide-trapping mechanism which pumps dietary I^- into the cell. The pump is very powerful, and the cell can concentrate iodide to 25–50 times its concentration in the plasma. Thyroid iodine content is normally around 600 μg/g tissue. *Uptake enhancers*: TSH; iodine deficiency; TSH receptor antibodies; autoregulation. *Uptake inhibitors*: I^- ions; cardiac glycosides (e.g. digoxin); thiocyanate (SCN^-); perchlorate ($PCl0_4^-$).

Inside the cell, I^- is rapidly oxidized by a peroxidase system to the more reactive iodine, which immediately reacts with tyrosine residues on a thyroid glycoprotein called thyroglobulin, to form mono-iodotyrosyl (T_1) or di-iodotyrosyl (T_2) thyroglobulin. These then couple to form tri-iodothyronine (T_3) or thyroxine (T_4) residues, still attached to thyroglobulin, which is stored in the colloid (i.e. $T_1 + T_2 = T_3$; $T_2 + T_2 = T_4$). This process is stimulated by TSH.

Under TSH stimulation, colloid droplets are taken back up

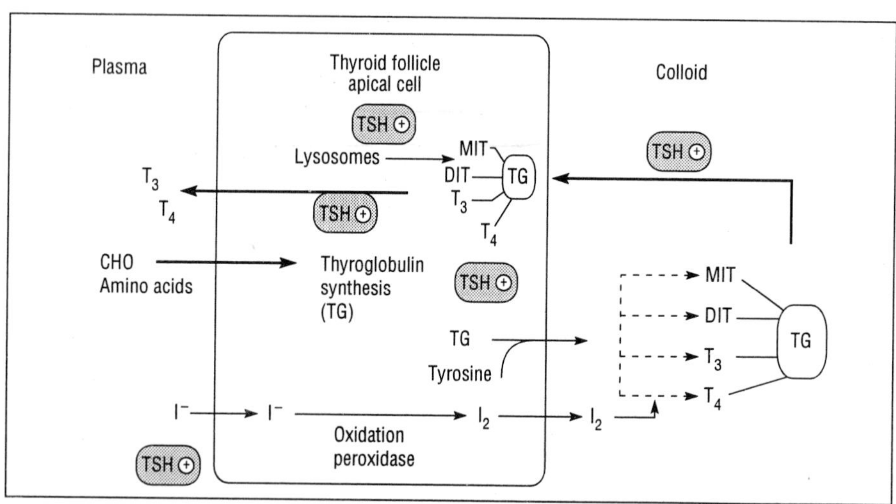

Fig. 9.2 Thyroid-hormone synthesis. TG, thyroglobulin; CHO, carbohydrate.

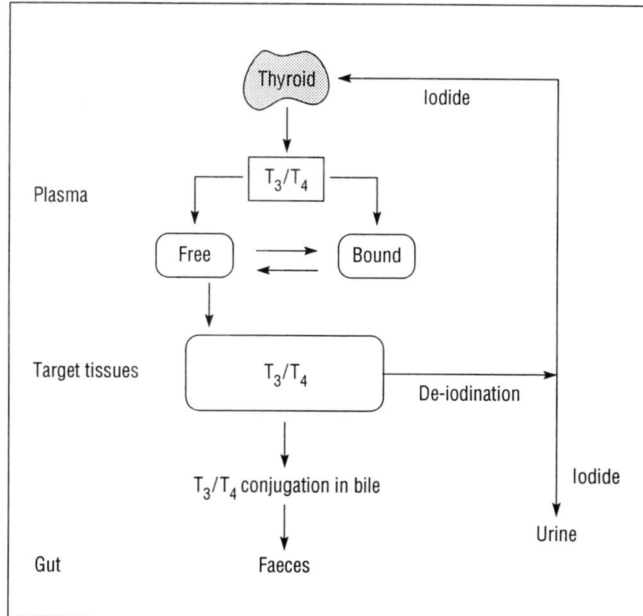

Fig. 9.4 Metabolism of thyroid hormone.

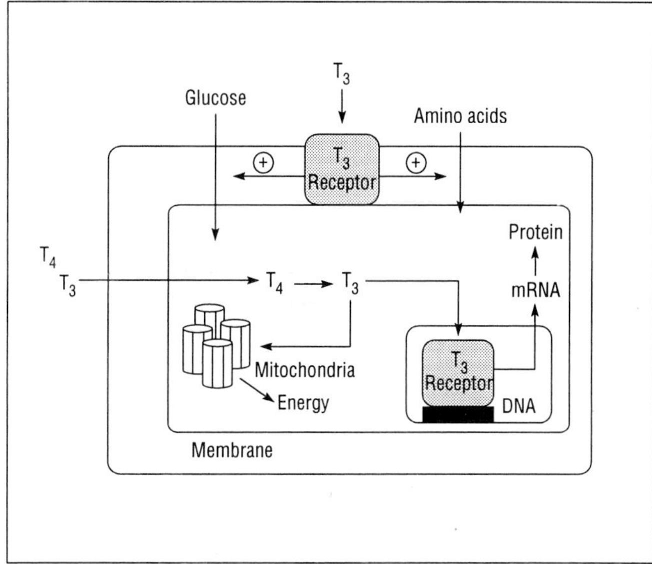

Fig. 9.5 Thyroid mechanism of action.

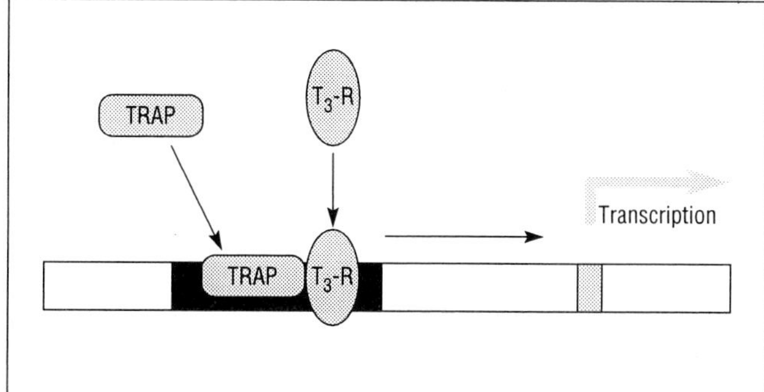

Fig. 9.6 Thyroid hormone-receptor action on target gene.

into the cell cytoplasm by micropinocytosis, where they fuse with lysosomes and are proteolysed to release the residues from the glycoprotein. T_1 and T_2 are rapidly de-iodinated by halogenases, and the liberated iodine is recycled in the follicle cell. Tri-iodothyronine and thyroxin are released into the circulation, where they are bound to plasma proteins, including thyroxin-binding globulin. Most is bound and therefore physiologically inactive, while only the free fraction is active.

Metabolism. The thyroid secretes a total of 80–100 μg of T_3 and T_4 per day, and the ratio of $T_4 : T_3$ is about 20 : 1. Although both T_3 and T_4 circulate, the tissues obtain 90% of their T_3 by de-iodinating T_4. Iodide liberated from thyroid hormone is excreted in the urine or is recirculated to the thyroid, where it is concentrated by the trapping mechanism. About one third of T_4 leaving the plasma is conjugated with glucuronide or sulphate in the liver and excreted in the bile. A small proportion of the free T_4 is reabsorbed via the enterohepatic circulation. The half-life of T_4 in the plasma is about 6–7 days; that of T_3 is very much shorter, being about 1 day. T_3 is much more potent than T_4.

Mechanism of action of thyroid hormone. There are multiple sites of action of T_3 in the cell. At the membrane, the hormone stimulates the Na^+/K^+–ATPase pump, resulting in increased uptake of amino acids and glucose, which causes calorigenesis (heat production). (*Note: earlier ideas that thyroid hormone produced heat by uncoupling oxidative phosphorylation have been disproved.*) T_3 combines with specific receptors on mitochondria to generate energy and with intranuclear receptors which are transcription modulators, resulting in altered protein synthesis. Thyroid receptor auxiliary protein (TRAP) stabilizes the T_3–receptor complex.

10 The thyroid: II

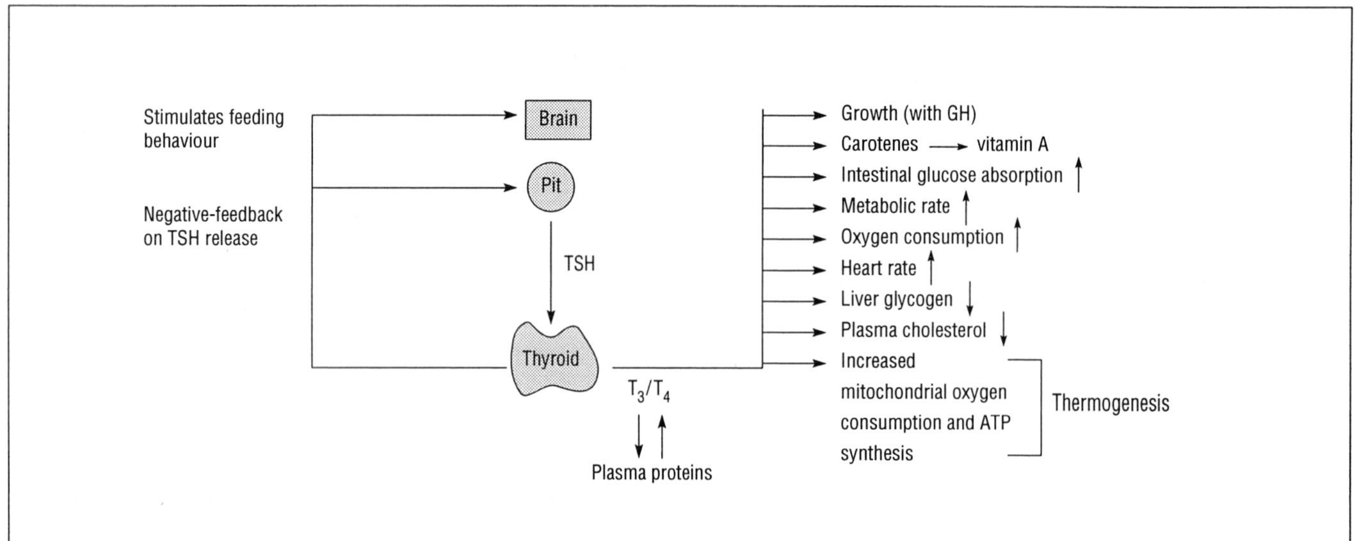

Fig. 10.1 Actions of thyroid hormone in mammals.

ACTIONS OF THYROID HORMONE

Calorigenesis. Homeotherms need to generate their own heat, and thyroid hormone does this by stimulating mitochondrial oxygen consumption and production of adenosine triphosphate (ATP) which is required for the sodium pump, which uses up to 40% of the total energy supply of the body. Cardiac glycosides such as ouabain, which blocks the Na^+/K^+–ATPase pump, inhibit the action of thyroid hormone.

Carbohydrate and fat metabolism. Thyroid hormone is catabolic: (i) stimulating intestinal absorption of glucose; (ii) stimulating hepatic glycogenolysis; (iii) stimulating insulin breakdown; (iv) potentiating the glycogenolytic actions of adrenaline. (*Note, however, that small doses of T_4 increase hepatic glycogenesis, and thyroid hormone actually potentiates the hypoglycaemic action of insulin by increasing glucose uptake into muscle and adipose tissue.*) Thyroid hormone is strongly lipolytic, by both a direct action and by potentiating (some call it 'permitting') the actions of other hormones, such as glucocorticoids, glucagon, growth hormone and adrenaline. Thyroid hormone also increases oxidation of free fatty acids, which adds to the calorigenic effect. Thyroid hormone decreases plasma cholesterol by stimulating bile acid formation in the liver, which results in excretion in the faeces of cholesterol derivatives.

Growth and development. In humans, little if any T_3 or T_4 passes from the maternal to the fetal circulation. When the thyroid is differentiated and functional at 10–11 weeks' gestation, thyroid hormone becomes essential for normal differentiation and maturation of fetal tissues, although the hormone is not necessary for normal fetal growth. Therefore, human cretins have retarded brain and skeletal maturation, but normal birth weight. In the brain, thyroid hormone causes myelinogenesis, protein synthesis and axonal ramification. It may act, in part, by stimulating production of nerve growth factor. Thyroid hormone is essential for normal growth hormone (GH) production. In addition, GH is ineffective in the absence of thyroid hormone. In tadpoles, thyroid hormone stimulates metamorphosis, possibly by increasing hyaluronidase production.

Thyroid hormone and prolactin. Thyroid hormone may be required for the normal production of prolactin by the anterior pituitary gland. The two hormones appear to act together to produce normal development of the mouse mammary gland.

CONTROL OF THYROID HORMONE PRODUCTION AND RELEASE

Normally, hypothalamic thyrotrophin-releasing hormone (TRH) stimulates thyrotrophin (TSH) release from the anterior pituitary thyrotroph cell. TSH belongs to a family of glycoproteins sharing common alpha and specific beta subunits. (*Note: in some cases of cretinism, it was found that the patient produced inactive beta subunits of TSH.*) TSH stimulates thyroid hormone release, which feeds back to the pituitary to limit TSH release.

Hyperthyroidism. If the thyroid is stimulated, for example, by TSH receptor antibodies (termed LATS: long-acting thyroid stimulator), circulating T_4 concentrations will be high, and TSH concentrations very low. Clinical hyperthyroidism is termed

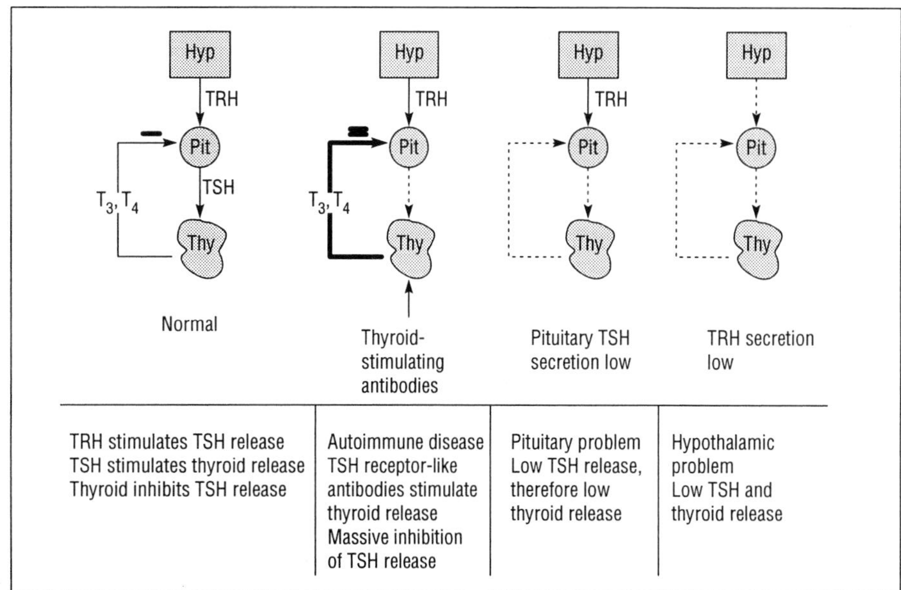

Fig. 10.2 Control of thyroid hormone.

thyrotoxicosis. Thyroid tumours may cause thyrotoxicosis. Graves' disease is the most frequent form of thyrotoxicosis, characterized by diffuse goitre (swollen neck), exophthalmos (protruding eyeballs) and a localized dermopathy of the leg with infiltration (oedema). The aetiology of Graves' disease is unknown, although it appears to be an autoimmune disease, genetically determined, and more frequent in women. Treatment for thyrotoxicosis involves reducing the release of thyroid hormone in order to achieve a euthyroid (normal) state. Treatment is by: (i) administering antithyroid drugs such as *thiouracil* (which blocks the peroxidase system); or by (ii) ingesting radioactive iodine to cause destruction of the tissue; or by (iii) surgical subtotal ablation of the gland.

Hypothyroidism can result from: (i) pituitary lesions, such as pituitary tumours; (ii) insufficient synthesis of thyroid hormone due to destruction of thyroid tissue in thyroiditis, or through congenital lack of thyroid tissue; dietary lack of iodine; (iii) surgical or chemical 'overkill' in removing thyroid tissue. Insufficient thyroid hormone causes increased TSH release, resulting in compensatory stimulation of the thyroid follicles, and goitre. Hypothyroidism is treated by administration of thyroxin.

11 The thyroid: III

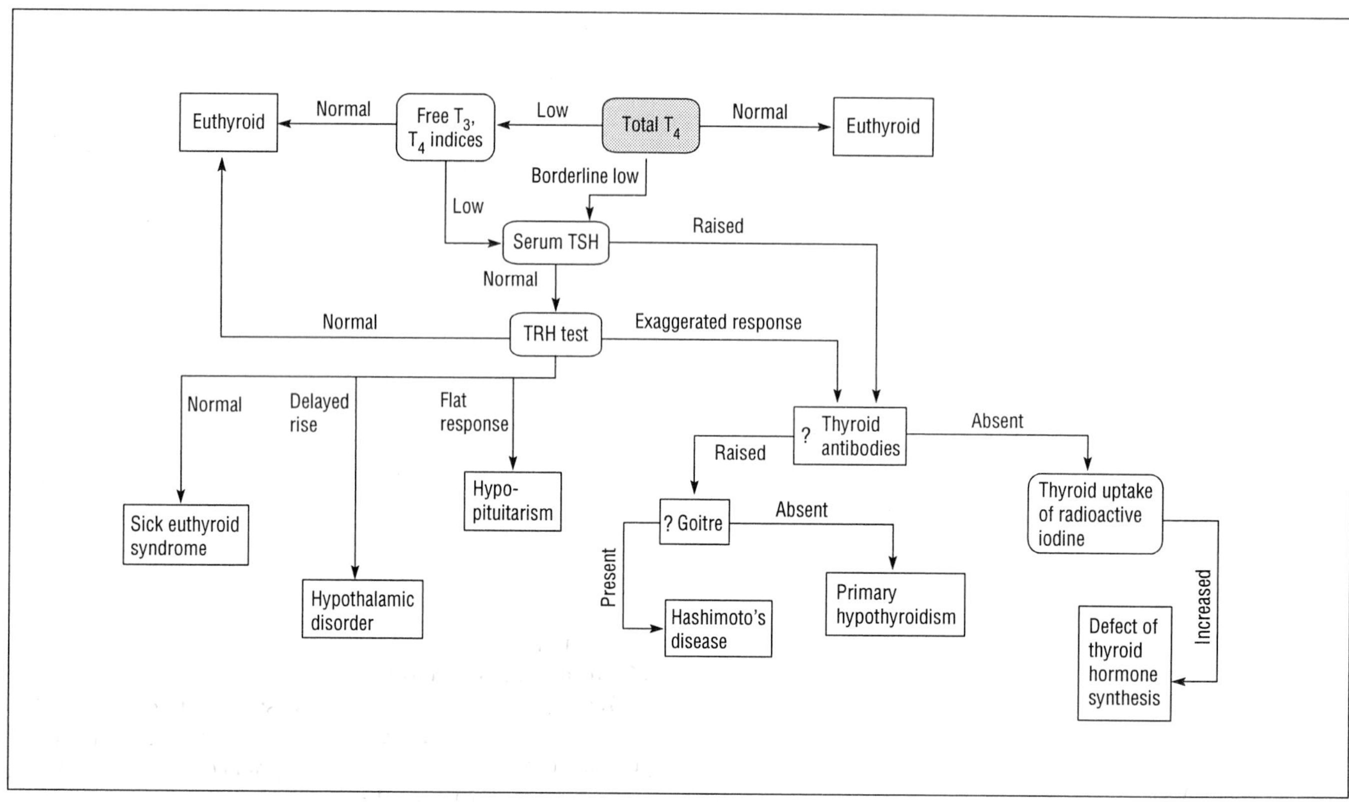

Fig. 11.1 Diagnostic tests for hypothyroidism.

DIAGNOSTIC TESTS FOR THYROID DISEASE

Hypothyroidism is characterized by: absent or very low levels of T_3 and T_4; low basal metabolic rate (BMR); loss of hair; facial oedema; coarse, dry skin and hair; patient complains of cold, due to decreased body temperature; intolerance to cold; decreased perspiration; slow pulse; tiredness; slow thinking processes; lethargy; sleepiness; weight gain; carotinaemia; irregularities of menstruation; goitre may occur.

Thyroid function tests have two aims: (i) to determine whether the patient is clinically hypothyroid; (ii) to localize the lesion(s) within the hypothalamic–pituitary–thyroid axis. T_3 and T_4 in plasma are assayed by radioimmunoassay (RIA: see page 18). The free hormone, which is the physiologically active form is also measured. The thyrotrophin-releasing hormone (TRH) test is a test of pituitary thyroid stimulating hormone (TSH) reserve, and of pituitary thyrotroph function. After administering TRH, both TSH and thyroid hormone levels in plasma should rise, if the pituitary responds to TRH. TSH may be administered to distinguish between primary hypothyroidism and other lesions in the axis. In primary hypothyroidism, plasma TSH is elevated and T_4 is low or undetectable. In Hashimoto's disease, in which the thyroid follicles are attacked by the immune system, similar hormone levels occur, together with goitre. (*Note: misleadingly low plasma levels of T_4 are found in non-thyroid related hypoproteinaemia caused by, for example, liver failure, nephrotic syndrome, or in familial deficiencies of plasma thyroxin-binding globulin.*)

Treatment. In patients without cardiovascular problems, thyroxin alone is given. TSH and T_4 are monitored and the dose of thyroxin adjusted to keep these in the normal range. If patients have angina, the thyroxin dose is lowered and given together with a beta blocker such as propranolol, unless the patient has congestive heart failure. Here, diuretics are given with T_3.

Hyperthyroidism. Excessive secretion of thyroid hormone can be due to a number of causes. It can be produced by excessive prescribing of thyroxin (iatrogenic), by excessive self-administration (thyrotoxicosis factitia), or from uni- or multinodular toxic goitre. It can also result from Graves' disease. Occasionally, hyperthyroidism may be produced by TSH secreted from hydatiform moles, embryonal testicular carcinomas or from choriocarcinomas, which produce a TSH-like material. TSH-secreting pituitary tumours are very rare.

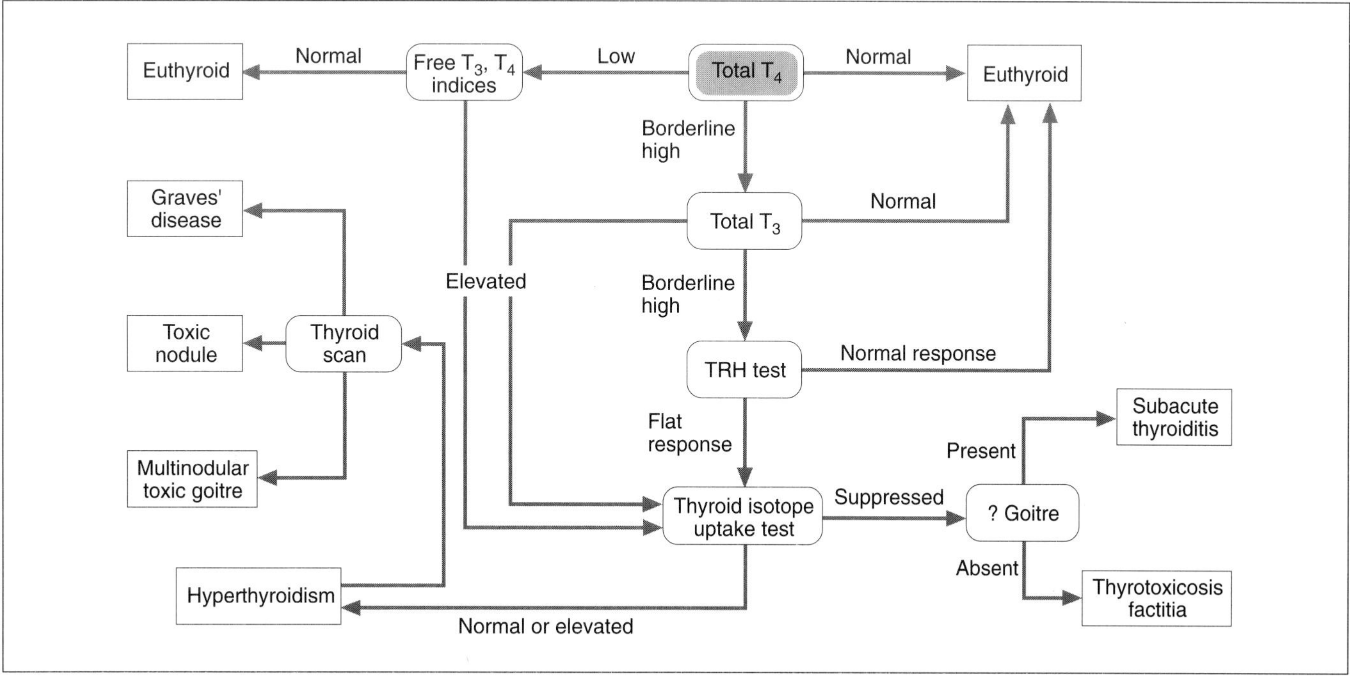

Fig. 11.2 Diagnostic tests for hyperthyroidism.

Misleadingly high plasma levels of T_3 and T_4 can occur in pregnancy and through the use of oral contraceptives, since oestrogens elevate thyroxin-binding globulin.

Hyperthyroidism is characterized by:

1 elevated levels of T_3 and T_4;
2 goitre;
3 increased BMR;
4 increased cardiac output and hypertension, causing rapid pulse;
5 increased perspiration;
6 intolerance to heat;
7 insomnia;
8 excitability;
9 nervousness;
10 irritability;
11 occasional exophthalmos;
12 weight loss;
13 sweaty palms;
14 irregularities of menstruation.

Treatments (i) antithyroid drugs, such as thiouracil, carbimazole, or its active metabolite methimazole, which inhibit the peroxidase system. In addition, propranolol may be given to counteract sweating, raised pulse and anxiety;
(ii) surgery, to perform partial thyroidectomy. Patients should be made euthyroid (normal thyroid blood levels) before surgery, as this reduces the risk of operative shock;
(iii) radioiodine therapy with ^{131}I, which destroys thyroid cell function. Like non-radioactive iodine, it is taken up preferentially by the thyroid through the trapping mechanism. Response is slow and patients need supplementary therapy with antithyroid drugs.

12 The adrenal gland: I

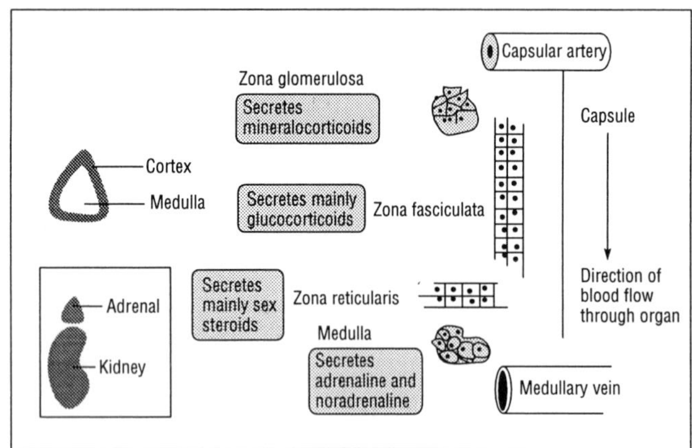

Fig. 12.1 Cellular organization in the adrenal gland.

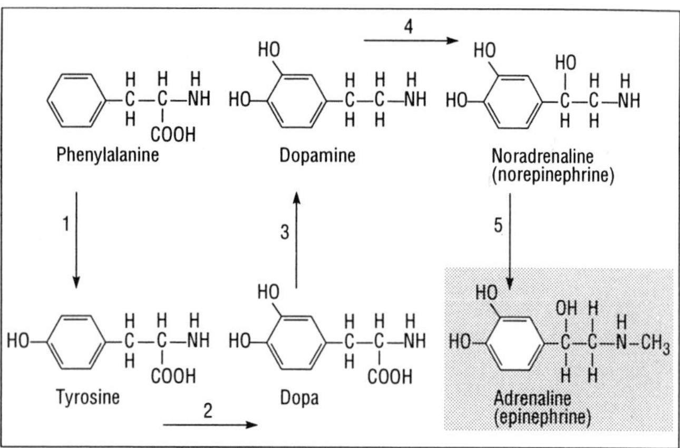

Fig. 12.2 Adrenaline synthesis.

THE GLAND

The adrenal gland lies just above the kidneys, and can be divided on anatomical and functional grounds into two main sub-organs: the adrenal cortex, which secretes the steroid hormones; and the adrenal medulla, a modified ganglion, which secretes the catecholamines adrenaline (epinephrine) and noradrenaline (norepinephrine).

ADRENAL MEDULLA

Catecholamine synthesis. The adrenal medullary chromaffin cells can be distinguished as adrenaline (AD)-storing and noradrenaline (NA)-storing cells. The enzymes catalysing synthesis are:

1 phenylalanine hydroxylase;
2 tyrosine hydroxylase, the rate-limiting step;
3 L-aromatic acid decarboxylase;
4 dopamine beta-hydroxylase;
5 phenylethanolamine *N*-methyltransferase (PNMT).

The catecholamines AD and NA are stored in the cell in granules, together with a protein, chromogranin, and adenosine triphosphate (ATP). When exocytosed, the granule releases all its contents.

Metabolism. Catecholamines are metabolized extracellularly and in the liver by catecholamine-*O*-methyltransferase (COMT), and intracellularly by monoamine oxidase (MAO). MAO is localized close to the adrenoceptors where AD and NA act. Catecholamine action is not terminated by enzymes, however, but through re-uptake into the cell from which they were released. Vanillylmandelic acid (VMA) is excreted in the urine. In sympathetic nerves, NA feeds back onto presynaptic alpha-2 receptors, which limit further release of NA.

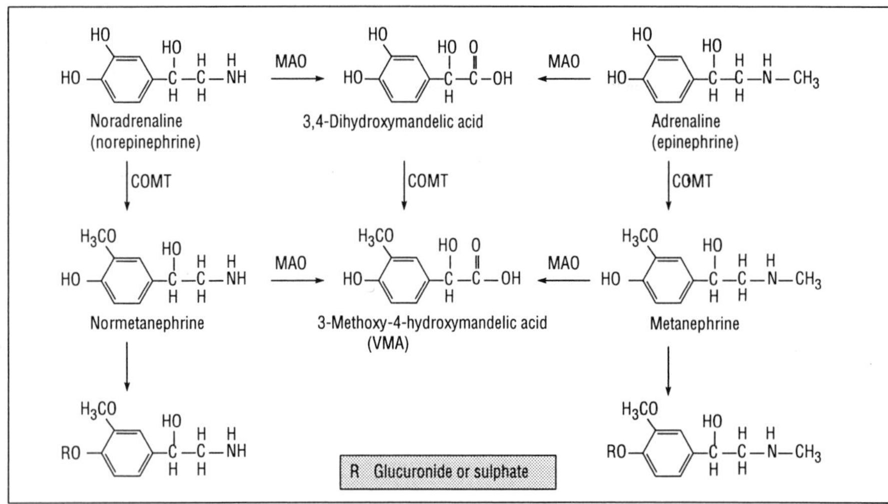

Fig. 12.3 Catecholamine catabolism.

ACTIONS OF ADRENALINE

Adrenaline has been called the hormone of 'flight or fight'. Stressors cause an immediate release of AD, which prepares the body for extraordinary physical and mental exertion. Surface vasculature shuts down by the constriction of arteriolar tissue through the mediation of alpha-1 receptors, thus limiting potential blood loss through injury; in contrast, the vasculature to the muscular beds opens up through the activation of the beta-2 receptors. Dilation of bronchioles increases the efficiency of oxygen intake in unit time, and glucose mobilization is enhanced through the stimulation of *glucagon* release and the inhibition of that of *insulin*. Dilation of the radial muscles increases the availability of light to the retina, and the contraction of the splenic capsule releases blood cells into the circulation. Through beta-1 receptors in the heart, contractility is greatly increased. AD also increases mental alertness, although the exact mechanism is unknown.

Mechanism of adrenaline action. An example of AD action is the mobilization of energy in the form of glucose. AD also acts on beta receptors in muscle to inhibit release of amino acids, thus reducing the rate of muscle proteolysis. This mechanism may be important in the fight or flight response, when muscle would be spared from providing energy. Although little NA is released from the adrenal medulla, it is the major neurotransmitter of the sympathetic nervous system which is activated during fight or flight.

Tissue	Effect	Receptor
Heart	Rate and force of contraction increased	Beta-1
Blood vessels	Skin, Mucous membranes, Splanchnic bed: Contract	Alpha-1
	Skeletal muscle: Dilate	Beta-2
Respiratory system	Bronchodilation	Beta-2
Gastrointestinal tract	Smooth muscle: Relax	Alpha-2
	Sphincters: Contract	Alpha-1
Blood	Coagulation time: Decreased	
	Red blood count [Haemoglobin], Plasma protein: Increased	
Metabolism	Insulin release: Decreased	Alpha-2
	Glucagon release: Increased	Beta-2
Eye-radial muscle	Contract	Alpha-1
Smooth muscle: Splenic capsule, Uterus, Vas deferens	Contract	Alpha-1

Fig. 12.4 Actions of adrenaline.

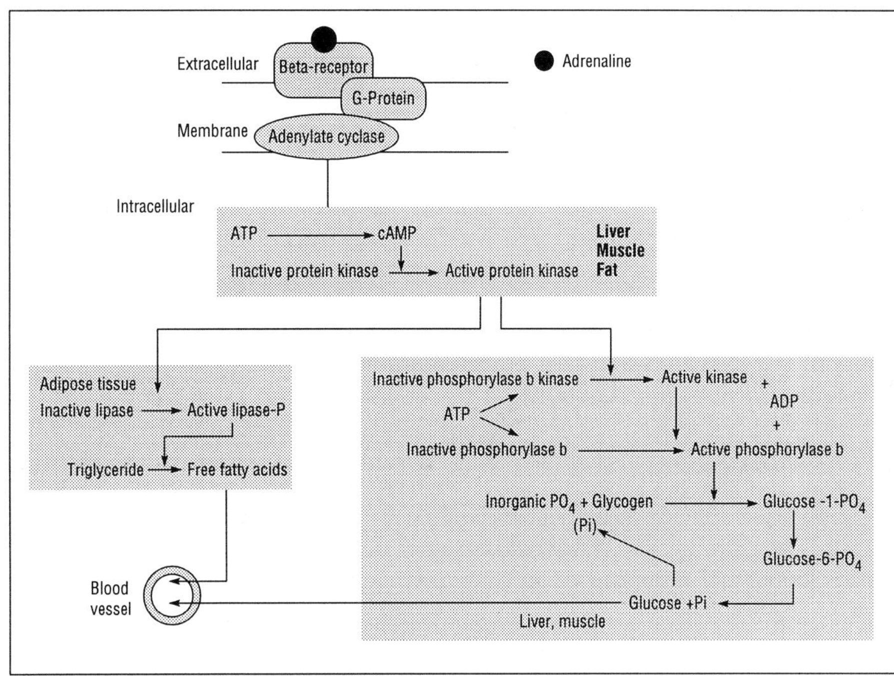

Fig. 12.5 Adrenaline action.

13 The adrenal gland: II

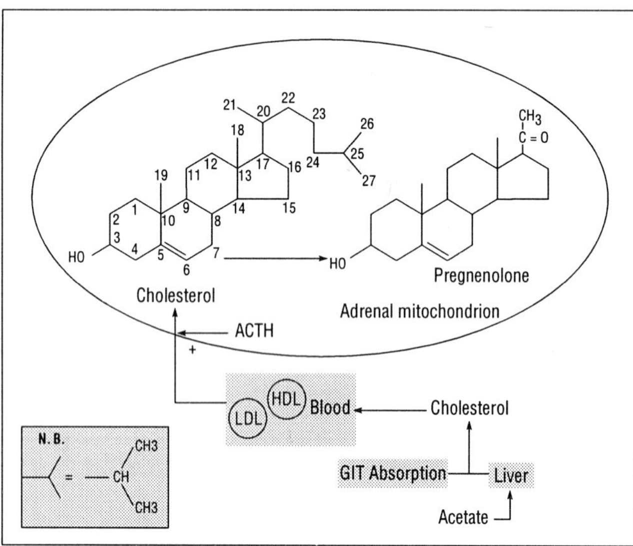

Fig. 13.1 Pregnenolone synthesis.

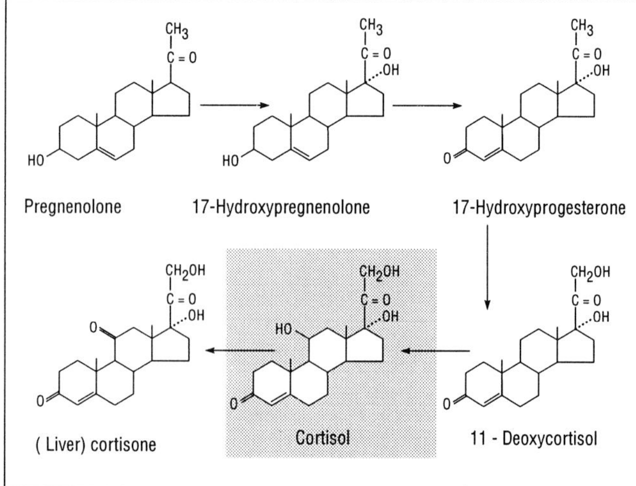

Fig. 13.2 Biosynthesis of adrenal glucocorticoids.

PREGNENOLONE SYNTHESIS

Pregnenolone is formed from cholesterol (CH) by side-chain cleavage catalysed by the desmolase enzyme system. CH is mainly transported in the blood in LDL (low density lipoprotein). Contrary to what was previously believed, most of the cell's CH is obtained from the bloodstream and not by intracellular synthesis. The LDL consists of an inner hydrophobic core of CH esters and triglyceride, surrounded by a monolayer of polar phospholipid and apoproteins. One of the apoproteins, apolipoprotein-E (APO-E), binds to receptors ('LP receptors') on the plasma membrane of the adrenal cell, resulting in an adrenocorticotrophic hormone (ACTH)-stimulated transport of CH into the cell. This sequence of actions is currently termed the LDL receptor pathway.

LDL has been linked with atherosclerotic disease, and the genetic disorder known as type III lipoproteinuria, associated with premature atherosclerotic disease, possibly occurs because of the nature of the APO-E in these individuals. Their APO-E does not bind with normal affinity to the LP receptor.

BIOSYNTHESIS OF GLUCOCORTICOIDS

After pregnenolone is released from the mitochondria, it is further metabolized in the smooth endoplasmic reticulum, where the double bond is switched from position 5 in the B ring to position 4 in the A ring, and the hydroxyl (OH) group at position 3 is oxidized to a keto group. Cortisol is formed through hydroxylation at the 11 position. Cortisol is the major glucocorticoid in humans, although further metabolism to another glucocorticoid, cortisone, occurs in the liver. (*Note that in the rat, a frequently used experimental animal in endocrine research, the major glucocorticoid is corticosterone.*)

SYNTHESIS OF ADRENAL ANDROGENS

Adrenal androgens are biosynthesized from androstenedione, which is formed from 17-hydroxyprogesterone by the cleavage of the C17 side chain, and hydroxylation at C17. Androstenedione, an adrenal androgen, can be formed through isomerization at the C4-C5 positions, as described previously for glucocorticoids, or after cleavage at C17. (*Note that for testosterone, the major androgen of the testis to be formed, there would have to be hydroxylation at the C17 position, but the enzyme that catalyses this is not present in high concentrations in the adrenal cell.*)

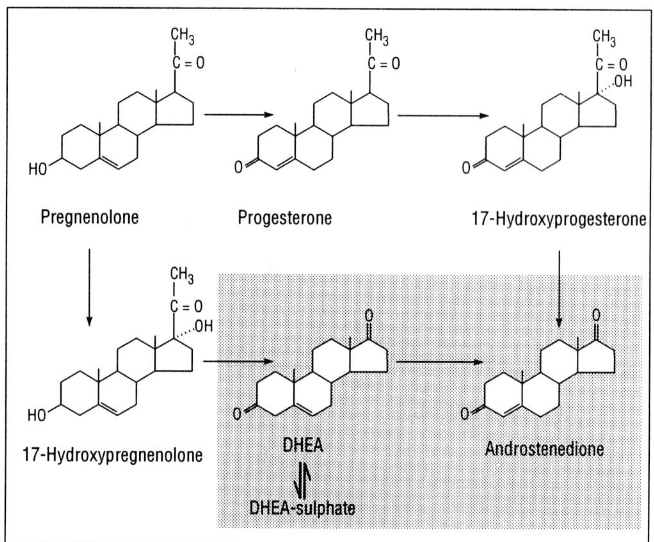

Fig. 13.3 Biosynthesis of adrenal androgens.

SYNTHESIS OF ADRENAL OESTROGENS

Oestrogens are formed from testosterone and androstenedione by aromatization of the A ring. The term 'aromatization' refers to the formation of alternating double bonds in the six-membered ring. The conversion is achieved through the removal of the methyl group at C19, and further oxidation. (*Note that testosterone gives rise to oestradiol, while androstenedione (not shown) gives rise to the oestrogen oestrone.*)

Neither the adrenal androgens nor the oestrogens are produced in sufficient quantities to support reproductive function; the testis and ovary, respectively, are required for that purpose, but adrenal androgens and oestrogens, and particularly the former, do become pathologically significant if produced in too high a concentration (see page 40).

The hormones are not stored, but are synthesized on demand, under the influence of the anterior pituitary hormone adrenocorticotrophic hormone (ACTH), which is the subject of the next section.

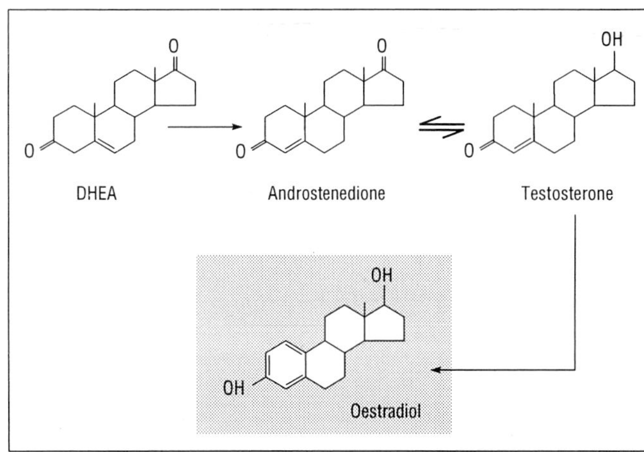

Fig. 13.4 Biosynthesis of adrenal oestrogens.

14 The adrenal gland: III

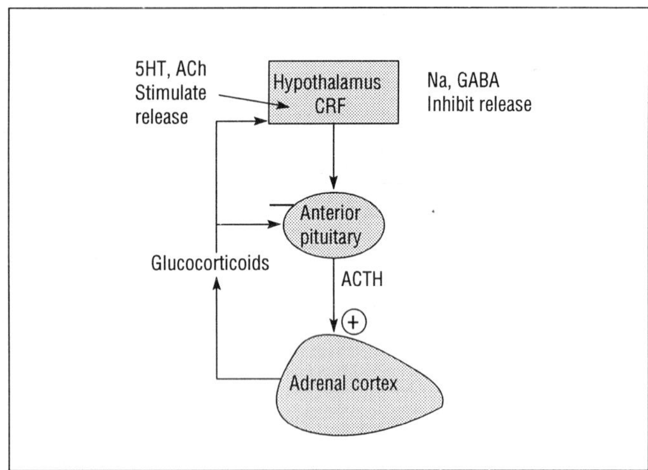

Fig. 14.1 Control of adrenal function.

ADRENOCORTICOTROPHIC HORMONE

Control of adrenocorticotrophic hormone (ACTH). ACTH is synthesized in the anterior pituitary corticotroph cells, and is released on stimulation of the corticotroph cell by the hypothalamic peptide corticotrophin-releasing hormone (CRF). Human CRF is a peptide containing 41 amino acids and is often referred to as CRF-41. It is a potent releaser of ACTH both *in vivo* and *in vitro*. CRF-41 is widely distributed throughout the brain, but the greatest concentration is in the hypothalamus, within the parvocellular neurones of the paraventricular nucleus (see page 22). These neurones project many fibres to the median eminence, where they release CRF into the portal circulation. Other peptides, notably vasopressin, may physiologically potentiate the ACTH-releasing action of CRF. The interaction between CRF and vasopressin (here abbreviated to AVP, because it is, structurally, arginine–vasopressin) involves their interaction with receptors on the membrane of the anterior corticotroph cell.

AVP activates the IP_3 second messenger system, which opens receptor-gated calcium channels. CRF, on the other hand, through the adenylate cyclase–cAMP second messenger system, opens voltage-gated calcium channels. The increased free intracellular Ca^{2+} stimulates ACTH release. ACTH synthesis is stimulated through CRF-mediated increased expression of the pro-opiomelanocortin (POMC) gene, which contains the genetic information required for synthesis of ACTH, and the hormone melanocyte-stimulating hormone (see below).

CRF release from the hypothalamus is stimulated by the neurotransmitters acetylcholine and 5HT (serotonin). It is inhibited by gamma-aminobutyric acid (GABA) and noradrenaline (NA). CRF and ACTH release are inhibited by the glucocorticoids in a negative-feedback loop, and this loop is most useful in testing the integrity of the hypothalamohypophyseal–adrenal axis. In principle, this is very similar to the tests of thyroid function (see page 28).

The pro-opiomelanocortin (POMC) system. Anterior pituitary corticotrophs synthesize a glycoprotein which contains the complete amino acid sequences of ACTH, beta-lipotrophin (beta-LPH), melanocyte-stimulating hormone (MSH), met-enkephalin and a number of other peptides. POMC has a 26 amino acid signal sequence, followed by three main structural domains, namely: (i) ACTH; (ii) beta-LPH at the C-terminal; and (iii) the N-terminal sequence (for which no biological role has yet been found). This sequence is termed pro-gamma-MSH. POMC is first cleaved to give beta-LPH and ACTH, which is still attached to the N-terminal fragment. In anterior pituitary corticotrophs, ACTH is released at the second cleavage. A

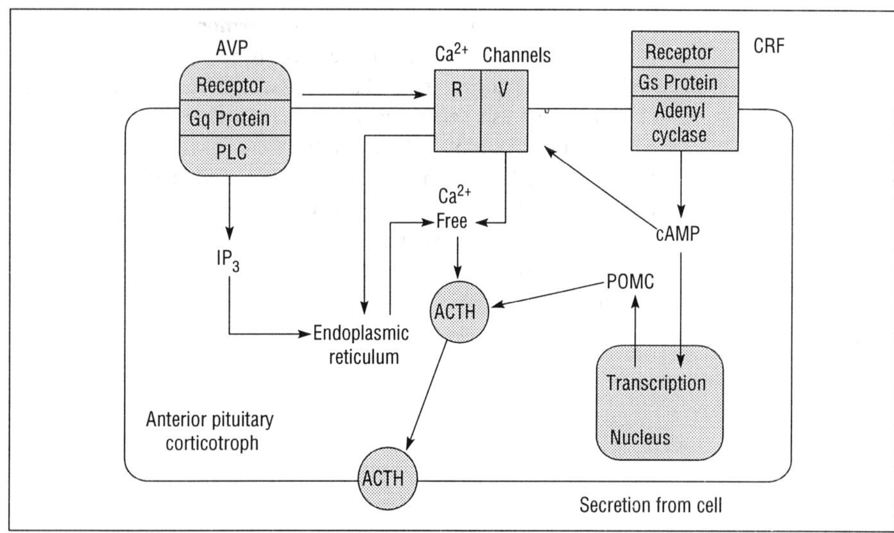

Fig. 14.2 Mechanism of action of corticotrophin-releasing hormone. R, receptor; V, voltage.

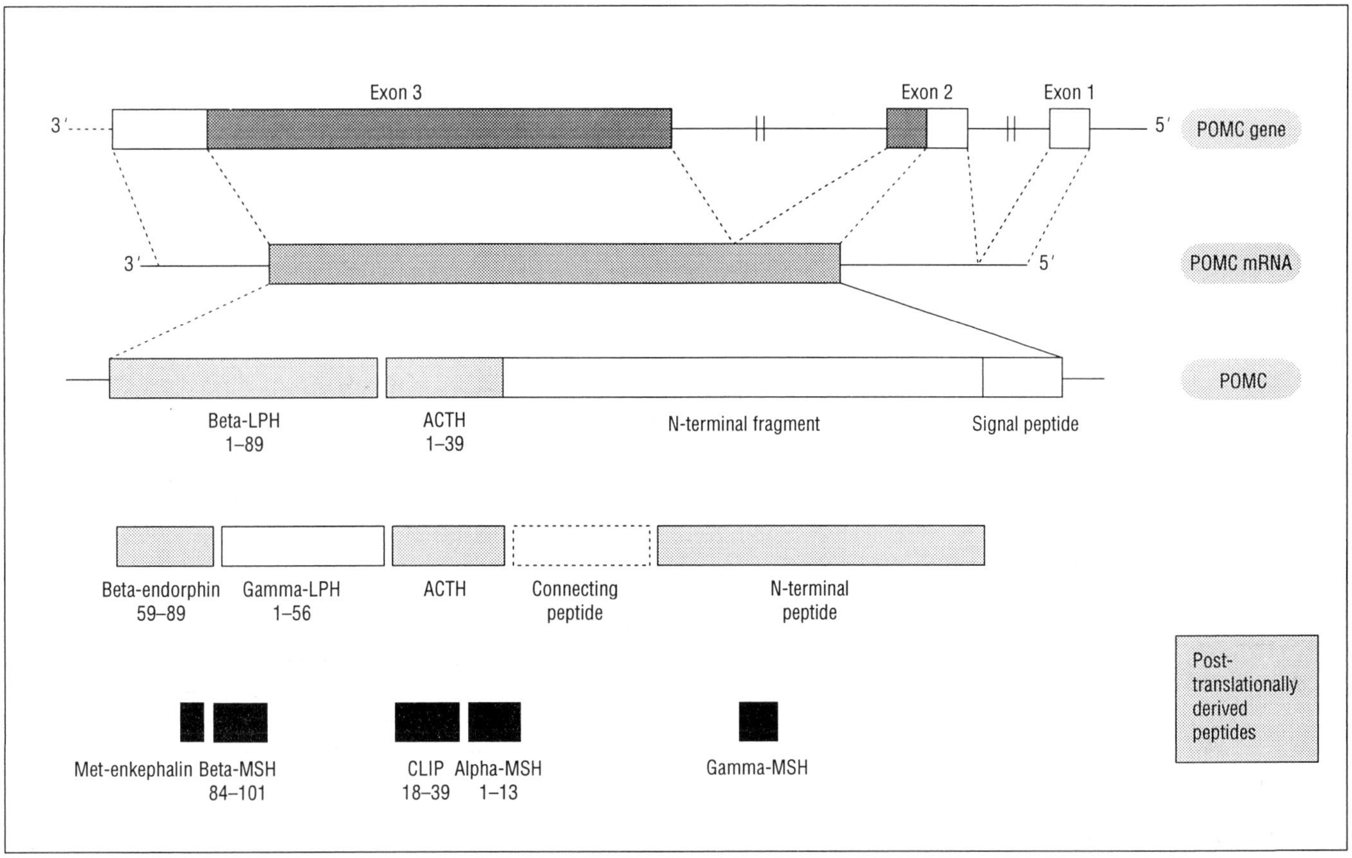

Fig. 14.3 The pro-opiomelanocortin system.

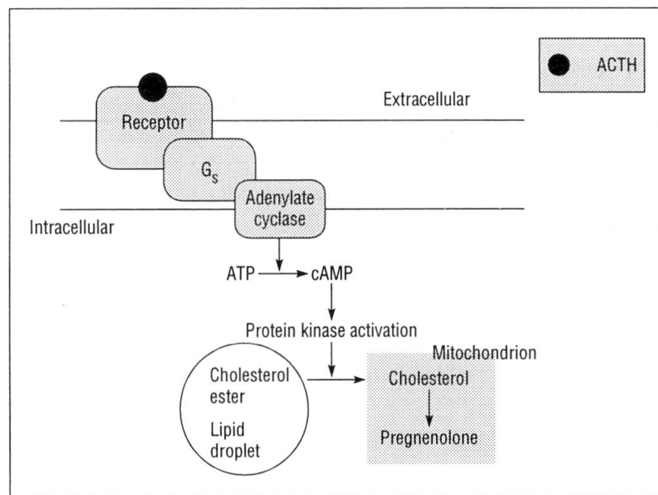

Fig. 14.4 Mechanism of action of adrenocorticotrophic hormone.

number of molecules of beta-LPH are cleaved to give beta-endorphin and gamma-LPH. It appears that on stimulation of the corticotroph with CRF, all the POMC-derived peptides are secreted together, suggesting thay they are held together in the same secretory granule, and supporting the idea that they all derive from POMC. In species which possess a pituitary intermediate lobe (e.g. the rat, but not the adult human), further cleavage of many of the peptides occurs: for example, the cleavage of ACTH into $ACTH_{1-13}$, which is alpha-*N* acetylated to yield alpha-MSH, and $ACTH_{18-39}$.

Mechanism of adrenocorticotrophic hormone action. ACTH binds to high affinity membrane receptors on the adrenal cell, activating the adenylate cyclase system. Maximum stimulation of steroidogenesis can be achieved with a plasma concentration of around 3 ng/l of ACTH. Increased intracellular concentrations of cAMP enhance the transport of cholesterol to a mitochondrial side chain cleavage enzyme, and they activate cholesterol ester hydroxylase. In addition, RNA and protein synthesis in the cell are stimulated, and there is a net increase in adrenal protein phosphorylation.

15 The adrenal gland: IV

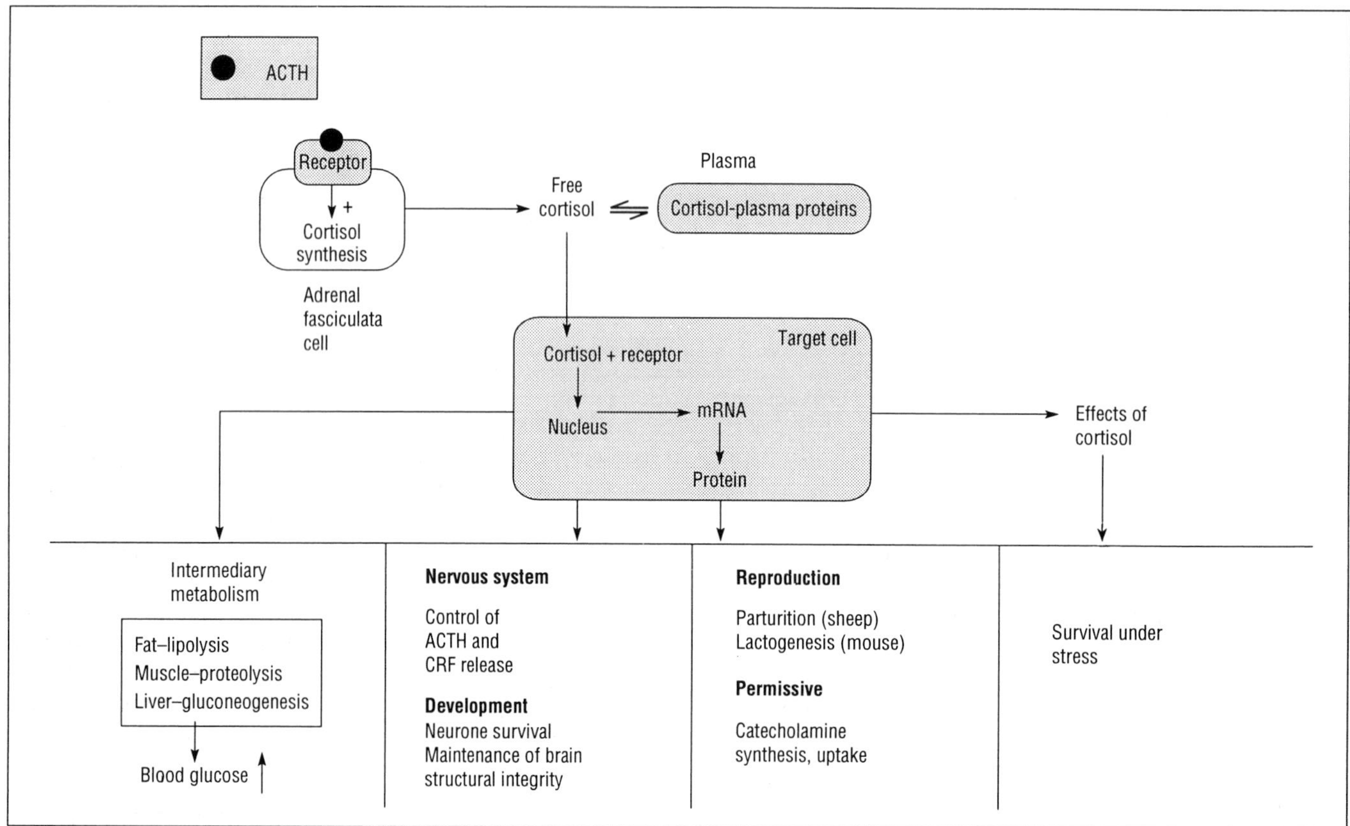

Fig. 15.1 Physiological actions of cortisol.

CORTISOL

Physiological actions of cortisol. Cortisol, like other steroid hormones, is poorly soluble in aqueous media, and after its release into the circulation, it is bound with high affinity by a plasma protein called, variously, transcortin, corticosteroid binding globulin or CBG. It is also bound with lower affinity by plasma albumin. Once bound, the steroid is physiologically inert, being unavailable to the target cells. Its half-life is extended, since it is also unavailable to the steroid-metabolizing enzymes of the liver. The free or unbound fraction (<10%) of the total plasma concentration is the biologically active form. (*The situation may be more complicated than this description suggests, since there is evidence that proteins which bind hormones themselves bind to target cells, and may even carry the hormone into these. At the moment, however, this is pure speculation.*)

Once inside the target cell, cortisol binds to cytoplasmic receptor proteins, and the complex is able to enter the nucleus and bind to target sites on the DNA upstream of the transcription initiation sites. As a result, mRNA and subsequent protein synthesis are affected. Physiologically, cortisol affects intermediary metabolism; the nervous system; and some processes related to reproduction. It permits other chemical mediators to act, and overall, it enables the organism to survive under stress.

Intermediary metabolism. Cortisol increases the synthesis of a number of enzymes which play key roles in hepatic gluconeogenesis. This is an anabolic action of cortisol. In adipose tissue (fat) and skeletal muscle, however, cortisol is catabolic, that is, it causes a breakdown of body tissues in order to mobilize energy. In these tissues, glucose uptake is inhibited, and another substrate for adenosine triphosphate (ATP) production is found through proteolysis in muscle and lipolysis in fat. The free fatty acids which are released from muscle and fat travel to the liver, where they are taken up and utilized as substrates for gluconeogenesis. The net result is increased glucose or hyperglycaemia.

Nervous system. Adrenocorticotrophic hormone (ACTH) and cortisol are synthesized and released in a diurnal (daily) rhythm (the term circadian is also used in rats and humans). The rhythm is determined by the interaction between the external environment, particularly the light–dark cycle and sleep patterns,

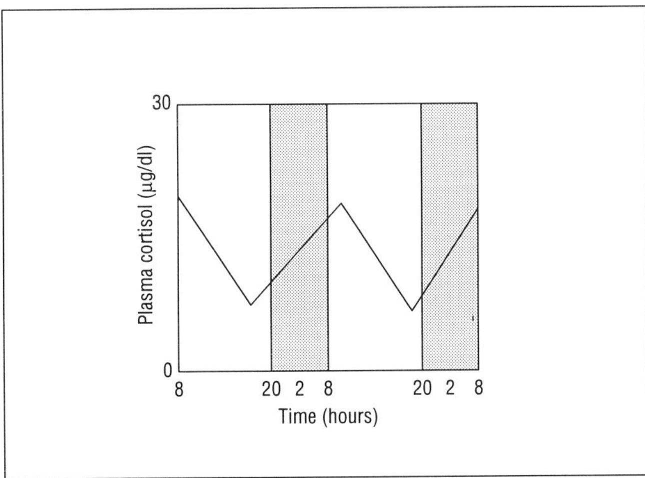

Fig. 15.2 Rhythm of cortisol release.

and this implicates the brain. The brain releases corticotrophin-releasing hormone (CRF), which in turn releases ACTH, which stimulates glucocorticoid release. Glucocorticoids feed back to the anterior pituitary and hypothalamus to limit ACTH and CRF release, respectively, through their intracellular receptors, and possibly through membrane glucocorticoid receptors. The application of the synthetic glucocorticoid dexamethasone abolishes the CRF stimulation of ACTH. The diurnal rhythm of glucocorticoid secretion reflects a similar rhythm of ACTH secretion. The rhythms are regulated by a 'biological clock', which may reside in the suprachiasmatic area of the brain (see page 22). The mechanism that causes the rhythm is thus inbuilt, but may be synchronized by exogenous (outside) influences such as light. This is particularly important in the case of seasonal breeding animals, where day length may determine the onset and offset of reproductive activity.

Glucocorticoids influence neuronal development in the fetal and neonatal brain. Administration of glucocorticoids to neonatal rats results in a reduction in both the basal level and the diurnal rhythm of ACTH and glucocorticoid release in the adult. This suggests that endogenous glucocorticoids may play a part in the normal development of the CRF–ACTH axis. In the adult rat, adrenalectomy (removal of the adrenal gland) results in the loss of neurones in specific regions of the hippocampus, an area of the brain concerned with memory, learning and the functioning of the hypothalamic–pituitary systems. Concurrent administration of glucocorticoids with adrenalectomy prevents neuronal loss, suggesting that glucocorticoids help to maintain cellular and structural integrity in specific areas of the brain.

Reproduction. Cortisol plays an important part in parturition (birth) in some species, notably the sheep. Plasma concentrations of cortisol rise in the fetal lamb some days before parturition, due to a mysterious increase in the sensitivity of the fetal adrenal cell to ACTH around a week before birth. In the mouse mammary gland, cortisol and prolactin are required for lactogenesis (milk production).

Permissive actions and stress. Glucocorticoids allow other hormones to exert certain effects. For example, they are required for catecholamine synthesis and re-uptake into nerve; they enable the process of catecholamine-stimulated fat mobilization and through their effects on gluconeogenesis, they permit the body to maintain its temperature and its response to stress. The body's response to stress has been termed the General Adaptation Syndrome (GAS). Three main phases have been postulated: (i) alarm reaction; followed by (ii) resistance; and then by (iii) exhaustion. The alarm reaction is the initial release of adrenaline from the adrenal medulla and the release of noradrenaline from sympathetic nerve terminals. At the same time, glucocorticoids are released, and these permit the catecholamines to act. Their onset of action is slower than that of the catecholamines, so they provide a continued resistance to stress. If stress is prolonged, this leads to exhaustion, characterized by muscle wasting, atrophy of tissues of the immune system, gastric ulceration, hyperglycaemia and vascular damage.

Table 15.1 Actions of glucocorticoids

Tissue	Action
Liver	Gluconeogenesis to increase glycogen stores
Fat	Lipolysis
Parturition	Fetal cortisol initiates parturition in sheep
Skeletal muscle	Atrophy through loss of protein
Connective tissue	Inhibition of growth
Immune system and lymphoid tissue	Suppression of immune system; atrophy of lymphoid tissue; mitosis inhibited; anti-inflammatory
ACTH	Inhibition of release from anterior pituitary gland
Water metabolism	Water retention by inhibiting glomerular filtration

16 The adrenal gland: V

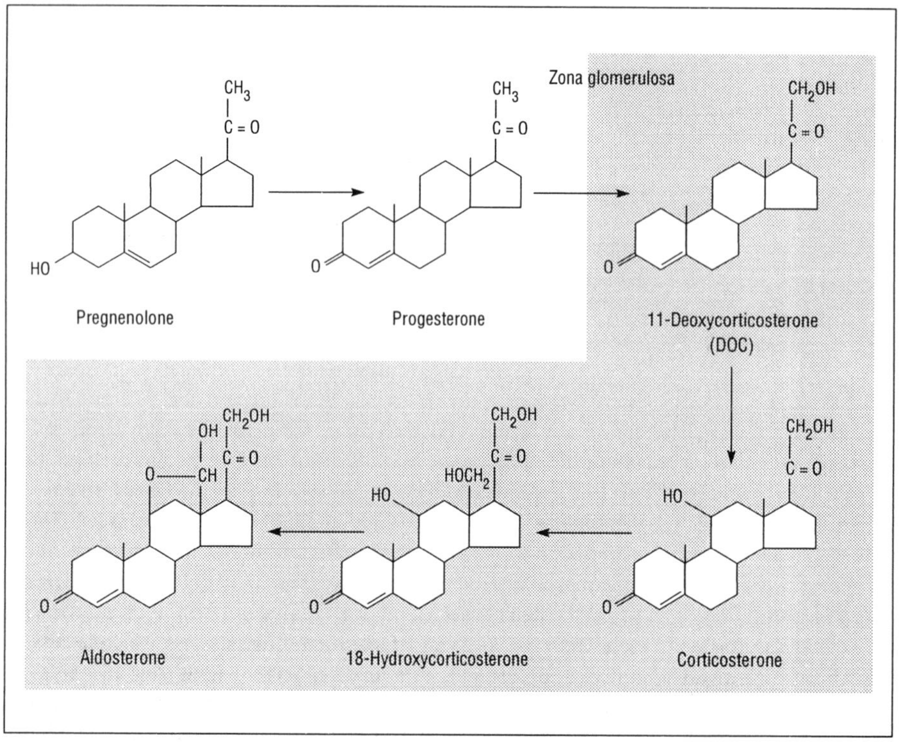

Fig. 16.1 Biosynthesis of aldosterone.

ALDOSTERONE

Aldosterone is the physiological mineralocorticoid (MC) of the body. In other words, it is an adrenal corticosteroid which affects cation concentrations and movements, specifically those of sodium and of potassium.

Deoxycorticosterone (DOC), a weaker MC, is also secreted. Both are synthesized in the zona glomerulosa, which lacks the enzyme 17-hydoxylase (see page 32). Progesterone is hydroxylated at C21 and C11-beta, resulting in corticosterone, which is hydroxylated at C18 and then oxidized to an aldehyde. This is shown as the last reaction product in what is called the haemiacetal form and is the form in which it is predominantly present. The secretion of aldosterone is controlled by the renin–angiotensin system (see page 72) and, to a lesser extent, by adrenocorticotrophic hormone (ACTH). Essentially, hyperkalaemia (raised blood K^+), ACTH, and angiotensin II can increase aldosterone release.

Mechanism of action of aldosterone. Aldosterone stimulates the active transport of sodium through the epithelial cell wall. Experimentally, aldosterone has been shown to stimulate the transport of Na^+ through amphibian (toad) bladder and skin. This action depends on protein synthesis. In common with the other steroid hormones, aldosterone stimulates *de novo* synthesis of proteins, which enhance sodium transport in the epithelial cell of the distal convoluted tubule of the kidney. The aldosterone receptor is also regulated by concentrations of aldosterone, higher concentrations of which reduce its production. Glucocorticoids bind, but with lower affinity than aldosterone, which explains their weak MC effect. Conversely, aldosterone binds weakly to glucocorticoid receptors, explaining its glucocorticoid effect when administered in high doses. The drug *spironolactone* competes with aldosterone for its receptor. There are three main theories to account for aldosterone action: (i) the hormone increases the number of sodium channels in the apical membrane; (ii) it increases the number of Na^+K^+-ATPase molecules; (iii) it increases adenosine triphosphate (ATP) molecule number within the cell. The hormone stimulates fatty acid synthesis and may alter membrane phospholipid composition as part of its mechanism of action.

Adrenal cortex pathophysiology. The symptoms of excess cortisol secretion (see Cushing's Disease, page 40) are similar to those of the side effects of prolonged glucocorticoid administration, for treatment of diseases such as rheumatoid arthritis. In fact, the symptoms have been termed Cushing's syndrome. Chronically increased plasma glucose (hyperglycaemia) stimulates excess insulin secretion. Eventually, the beta-cells of the pancreatic islets are exhausted and diabetes mellitis, also called steroid diabetes, results. The kidneys have to eliminate excess glucose, which drags solvent (water) with it, resulting in polyuria and polydipsia (excessive water drinking). This is to some extent counteracted by the weak MC effect of the glucocorticoids,

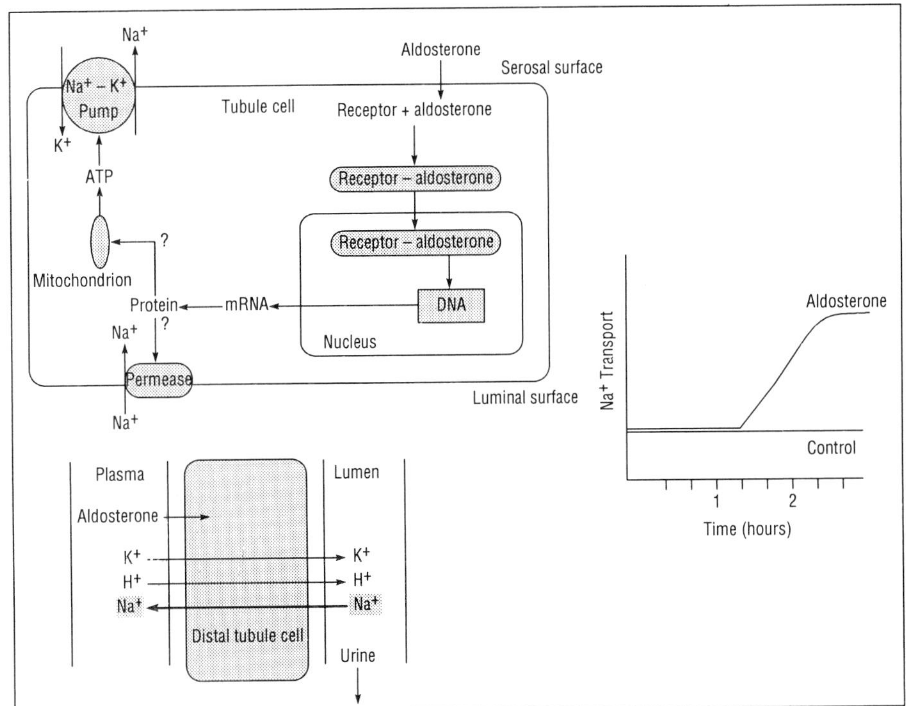

Fig. 16.2 Aldosterone action.

which may produce hypertension due to cation and water retention. The swollen ankles seen in patients on chronic glucocorticoid therapy reflects water retention. Patients on prolonged glucocorticoid therapy develop the characteristic 'moon face' and 'buffalo hump' due to redistribution of body fat. Both ACTH and glucocorticoids are lipolytic in normal fat stores, and the excess insulin may be lipogenic in the face, upper back and in the supraclavicular fat pads.

The catabolic effect of glucocorticoids on protein puts the body into negative nitrogen balance, with muscle wasting and weakness. The skin and subcutaneous tissues bruise easily, and there is thinning of skin and bones. Loss of bone protein matrix results in osteoporosis, with a tendancy for collapse of the thoracic and lumbar spine and for asymptotic rib fractures. Glucocorticoids suppress the immune system by atrophying lymphoid tissue and inhibiting lymphocyte function.

Prolonged treatment with glucocorticoids drives down ACTH release, therefore endogenous corticol production is extremely low. Thus, patients have to be weaned off glucocorticoids slowly to allow the rise of plasma cortisol to normal levels.

17 The adrenal gland: VI

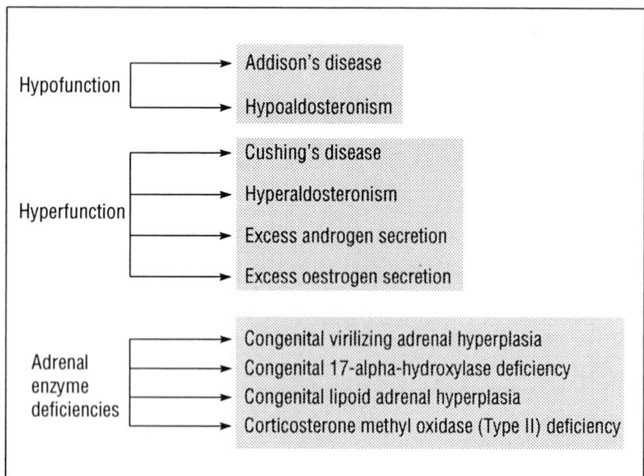

Fig. 17.1 Pathophysiology of the adrenal cortex.

HYPOFUNCTION

Addison's disease. First described by Addison in 1855, the disease is caused by the destruction of adrenal tissue. Before World War II, it was predominantly caused by tuberculosis, but now occurs through idiopathic (unknown cause) destruction of the adrenal cortex. The disease may be autoimmune, since adrenal autoantibodies are detected in the plasma of many patients. The disease sometimes presents first as an Addisonian crisis, with fever, abdominal pain and hypotensive collapse and pigmentation of skin and mucous membranes, due to very high circulating concentrations of adrenocorticotrophic hormone (ACTH) and related pituitary-derived peptides, such as melanocyte-stimulating hormone (MSH). Areas often affected include the skin under the fingernails, labia, scrotum, nipples and buccal mucosa. The diagnosis is confirmed using the ACTH stimulation test. The patient is injected intramuscularly with a synthetic fragment of ACTH, which contains the first 24 amino acids of the natural peptide, and plasma cortisol is measured. In patients with a non-responsive adrenal gland, plasma cortisol will be low.

The presence of adrenal autoantibodies, and of tubercular calcification of adrenal tissue (detected using X-ray) may be included as adjuncts to the ACTH stimulation test. There is, also, hyperkalaemia, hyponatraemia (low blood sodium) and high urine Na^+. Initial treatment, if the patient is in crisis, is intravenous saline solution to correct low blood volume, and hydrocortisone. Thereafter, the patient is maintained on oral glucocorticoids, for example, *prednisolone* and a synthetic mineralocorticoid (MC) such as *fludrocortisone*.

Adrenal insufficiency may be secondary to diseases of the hypothalamohypophyseal axis. A pituitary tumour may cause decreased secretion of ACTH and other peptides, such as MSH, when the symptoms of Addison's disease will be observed, but not the hyperpigmentation.

Hypoaldosteronism, which is a deficiency of aldosterone release resulting in sodium loss, occurs in the following.
1 Addison's disease (see above), or may be due to hypopituitarism, or to specific enzyme deficiencies (see below).
2 Diabetes, and may be secondary to deficient renin release. This may occur due to neuropathies (nerve damage) which affect the beta-adrenergic stimulation of renin release from the kidney. Patients with hypoaldosteronism, as a consequence of reduced renin secretion, are said to suffer from Conn's syndrome.
3 Very rarely, some patients are insensitive to their own aldosterone, perhaps because of an aldosterone receptor defect in the target cell.

HYPERFUNCTION

Cushings's syndrome, first described by Cushing in 1932, refers to the excessive secretion of glucocorticoids (see also page 38). Outlined below are four principal causes.
1 Primary hypercortisolism, due to an adrenal cortical tumour. The tumour may be an adenocarcinoma, which is a malignant epithelial tumour of glandular tissue, or a carcinoma, which may arise in any epithelial tissue, but which is not necessarily glandular. The symptoms are those of excess glucocorticoid in blood (see above), and very low or absent ACTH due to suppression of release by cortisol. The patient, therefore, has no ACTH-related pigmentation.
2 Drugs, such as ACTH or glucocorticoid treatment. Any drug-induced disease is said to be *iatrogenic*.
3 ACTH from an ACTH-secreting tumour, for example, an oat cell carcinoma of the lung, or tumours in the thymus or pancreas, or (rarely) in the ovary. These types are called the Ectopic ACTH syndrome. It is detected by marked hypokalaemia, which is rare in primary hypocortisolism.
4 Increased secretion of ACTH from the pituitary. This is Cushing's disease. It may result from a pituitary adenoma (about 75% of cases) or an hypothalamic defect.

Clearly, when ACTH is raised together with raised cortisol, this means the ACTH-secreting tissue is operating outside the negative-feedback mechanism, and if patients are injected with a synthetic glucocorticoid such as dexamethasone, this does not bring down plasma levels of ACTH.

Excess sex hormone secretion. Stimulation of the adrenal cortex by excess ACTH causes abnormal synthesis and release of sex hormones, particularly of androgens, which produce hirsutism in women. Of more importance in this respect, however, are the deficiencies of steroidogenic enzymes.

Congenital virilizing adrenal hyperplasia. This is a deficiency of

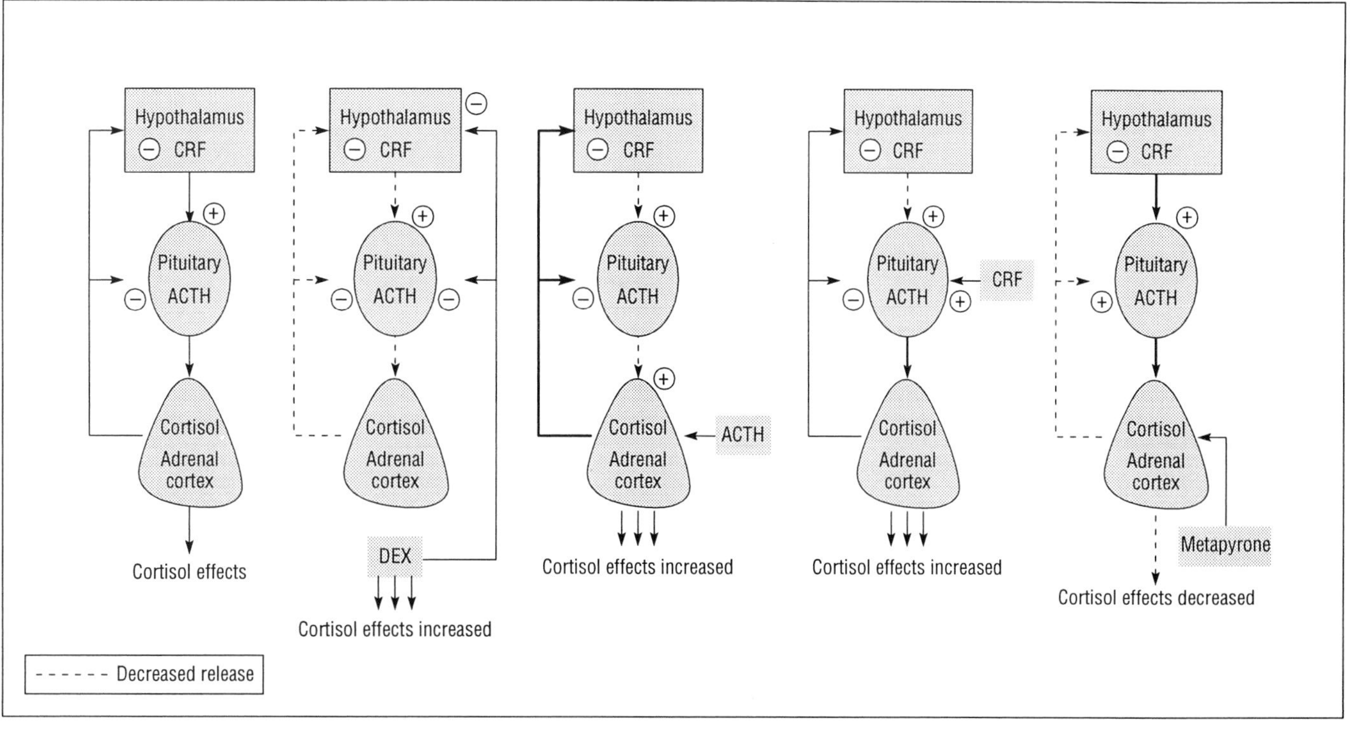

Fig. 17.2 Tests of adrenal axis function.

steroidogenic enzymes involved in cortisol and aldosterone production. There may be a deficiency of:

1 3-beta-hydroxysteroid dehydrogenase, which converts pregnenolone to progesterone, 17-hydroxypregnenolone to 17-hydroxyprogesterone, and dehydroepiandrosterone (DHEA) to androstenedione. Thus DHEA, an androgen, builds up and virilizes the newborn, which also has no salt-retaining facility. This congenital defect is usually fatal.

2 11-beta-hydroxylase, which converts 11-deoxycortisol to cortisol. Deoxycorticosterone and subsequent aldosterone synthesis are enhanced, producing hypertension. Increased androstenedione production causes virilization of both men and women.

3 21-beta-hydroxylase, which converts progesterone to 11-deoxycorticosterone and 17-hydroxyprogesterone (17-OHP) to 11-deoxycortisol. This results in increased synthesis of androgens due to increased availability of 17-OHP. The deficiency of aldosterone results in sodium and water loss.

All forms of the disease are treated with glucocorticoid replacement and MC, if necessary.

Congenital 17-alpha-hydroxylase deficiency. No 17-hydroxylated steroids can be formed, therefore little or no androgen or cortisol is produced, but aldosterone production is unimpaired. Because there is no glucocorticoid feedback to limit ACTH release, aldosterone production is driven up, resulting in hypertension. Treatment with dexamethasone inhibits ACTH release and at the same time removes the deficiency of glucocorticoid.

Congenital lipoid adrenal hyperplasia. This is a rare disease, caused by the deficient conversion of cholesterol to pregnenolone. The lack of cortisol feedback results in increased release of ACTH, which stimulates the adrenal cells to take up more cholesterol.

Corticosterone methyl oxidase (Type II) deficiency. In some families, there is a deficiency of the enzyme which oxidizes the hydroxyl (OH) group at position C18, which normally results in the aldehyde group. In affected individuals this results in hypoaldosteronism.

See page 102 for a summary of steroid pathways and enzymes.

Tests of adrenal axis function. Dexamethasone (DEX) administration should decrease ACTH release if the feedback mechanism is working, or if there is no autonomous ACTH-releasing tumour. ACTH administration should create increased cortisol production and release, if the adrenal gland is able to synthesize cortisol. Corticotrophin-releasing hormone (CRF) should stimulate ACTH release if the pituitary is able to respond to CRF. The effects of increased cortisol should be evident, and increased cortisol-derived metabolites measured in urine. *Metyrapone*, an inhibitor of cortisol production, is used to test the ability of the anterior pituitary to respond to decreased circulating cortisol by increasing its release of ACTH. Metyrapone, which acts by inhibiting 11-beta-hydroxylase, is useful in distinguishing Cushing's syndrome of ectopic origin, in which case administration of the drug will not affect the circulating concentration of ACTH.

18 Sexual differentiation and development: I

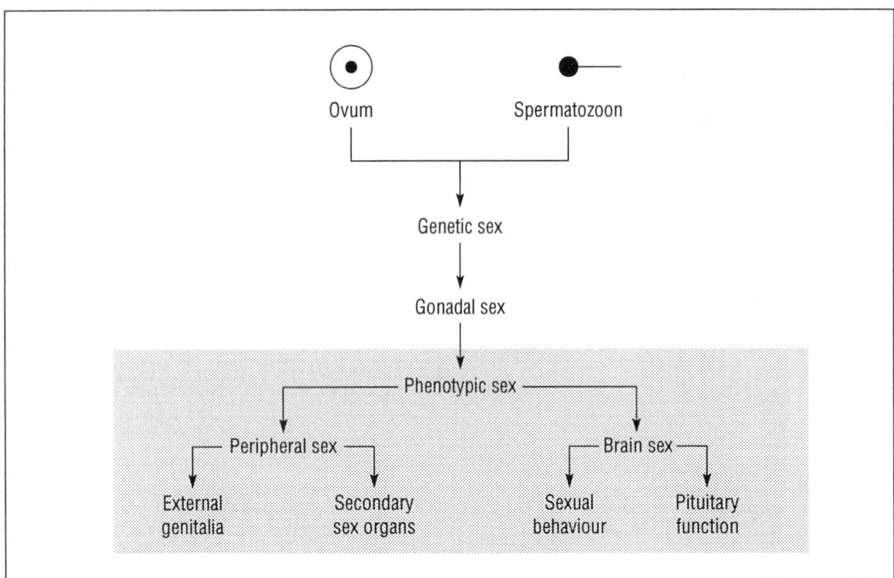

Fig. 18.1 Role of hormones in development.

Sexual differentiation can be classified according to: (i) the genetic sex of the phenotype, that is, whether it is XX (homogametic) or XY (heterogametic) with respect to the sex chromosomes, and (ii) according to the sexual characteristics determined by the gonadal hormones. Every human normally has 46 chromosomes in each cell, consisting of 22 pairs of autosomal chromosomes, and a pair of sex chromosomes. Genetic sex is determined at the time of conception, when male and female gametes, as the sperm and ovum are called, fuse to form a new individual. The possession of XX chromosomes means that a female will develop. It is now known that a Y chromosome determines that a male will develop.

The Y chromosome possesses what is termed the sex-determining gene, also called the *Sry* gene, which expresses the Sry antigen. This is a fairly recent discovery, and in older textbooks reference may be made to the H–Y antigen, which was thought to be responsible for the development of a testis, or male gonad. The situation with respect to testis development is not straightforward, however, since XX females can develop a testis. Therefore the Sry antigen is a trigger that switches on

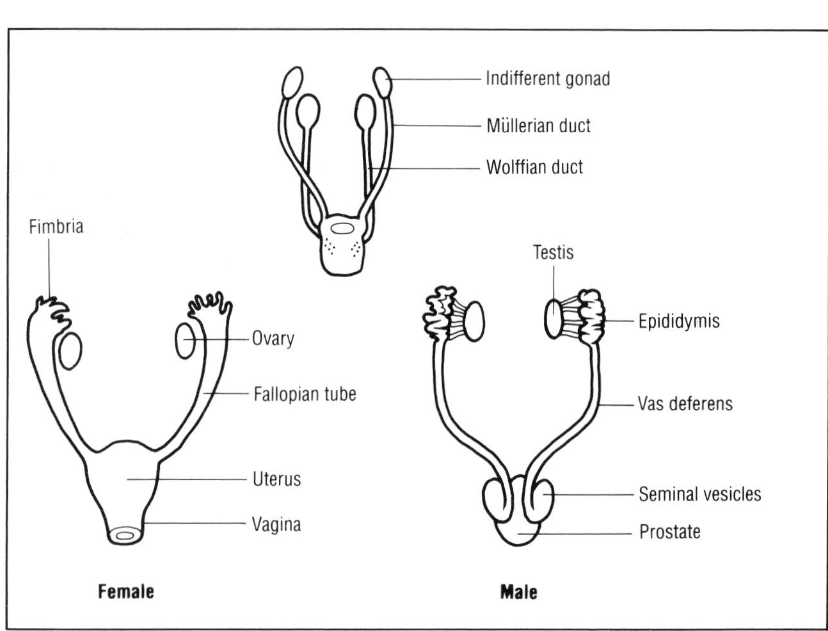

Fig. 18.2 Sexual differentiation of the reproductive organs.

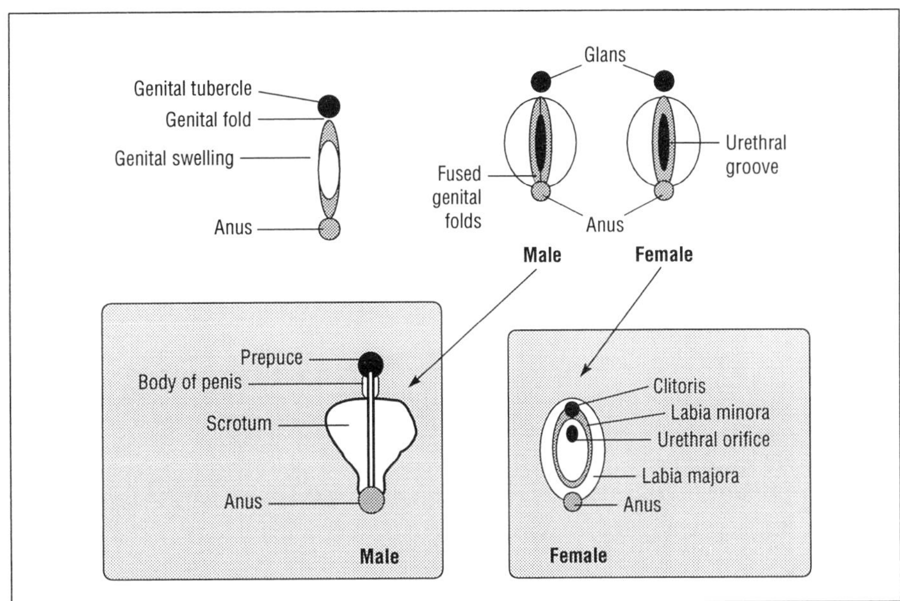

Fig. 18.3 Differentiation of external genitalia.

genes on other chromosomes responsible for testis development. The question about what determines gonadal sex cannot be answered until it is known what triggers Sry antigen expression.

GONADAL SEX

In the human fetus, at about 4 weeks, the gonads are indifferent, that is, they cannot be distinguished as testis or ovary, and are capable of developing into either. The indifferent gonad before differentiation is composed of a coating of germinal epithelium, the genital ridge mesenchyme, and the primordial germ cells. Thereafter, under the influence of the Sry antigen, the primordial germ cells will move to what is called the medullary region of the primitive gonad. Still under Sry influence, the indifferent gonad begins to develop into a testis. Primitive sex cords give rise to the seminiferous tubules, whose lining of epithelial cells will differentiate into the germinal epithelium, which will give rise to the spermatogonia and the Sertoli cells, which appear to nourish growing spermatids (see page 63). These epithelial cells also differentiate into the Leydig cells, which will produce the male sex hormone testosterone.

Where the seminiferous tubule leaves the testis, it branches extensively to form the rete testis, which transports the sperm to the tubules. In the absence of the Sry antigen, the ovary develops. The ovary develops later than does the testis, although both gonadal forms develop steroidogenic competence at the same time. Thus the ovary can synthesize oestrogens when the testis can synthesize testosterone, although it is not known whether oestrogens are important in the development of the female fetus.

PHENOTYPIC SEX: PERIPHERAL SEX

Ductal differentiation. Before differentiation, the ductal systems are bipotential: either can develop. If a testis develops, it produces a Müllerian regression factor, also known as anti-Müllerian hormone (AMF). AMF is a glycoprotein of molecular weight of about 70 KDa, which causes atrophy of the Müllerian ducts. The testis Leydig cells also start to secrete testosterone, which supports the development of the Wolffian ducts. This in turn leads to the development of the epididymis, seminal vesicles and the ductus deferens. In the absence of the ovaries and testis (i.e. if they are removed from the developing fetus, or not functioning), the Müllerian ducts develop and the Wolffian ducts wither, which suggests that the gonads are not required for the development of a female ductal system.

External genitalia. In the absence of the Y chromosome, the female phenotypical external genitalia will develop. When the fetal testis starts producing androgen, the penis and scrotum form and the testes descend. In the female, the genital tubercle will become the clitoris and the labia will develop.

19 Sexual differentiation and development: II

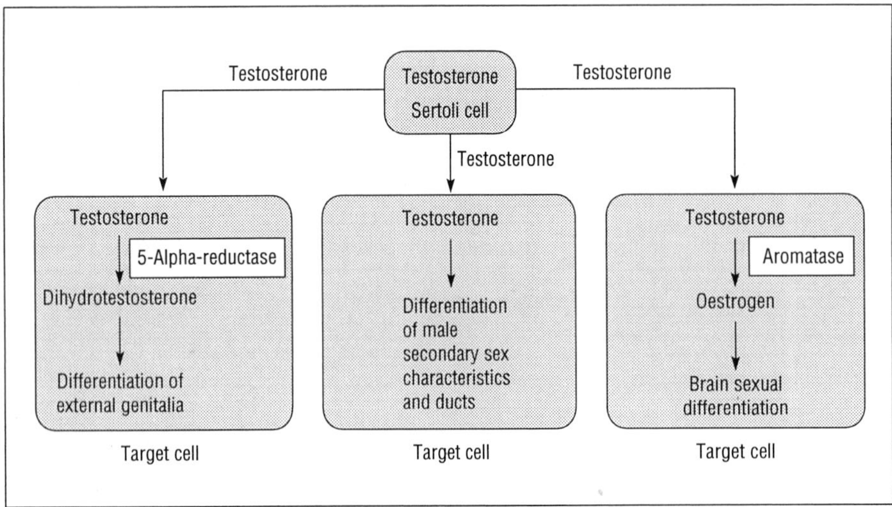

Fig. 19.1 Sexual differentiation.

PHENOTYPIC SEX: BRAIN SEX

This is a controversial area of endocrinology. From experiments with rodents, it appears that the brain is, like the rest of the body, inherently female, unless the Sry antigen intervenes to form a male gonad or testis, which produces androgen. In the periphery, androgens form the male external genitalia after reduction to the metabolite dihydrotestosterone (DHT).

In the brains of rodents, androgens alter the development of specific brain nuclei, particularly in the hypothalamus, which mediate sexual behaviour and gonadotrophin release. In the rat, the preoptic area of the male (see page 22) is far larger than that of the female, due to the perinatal actions of sex hormones on this brain area. Unlike the situation peripherally, androgen produces its differentiating effects through local conversion in the brain to oestrogens. These combine with oestrogen receptors to alter the size of certain nuclei or groups of brain cells. There is evidence that a similar mechanism may operate in primates, including humans.

Sex hormones may differentiate the human brain from about 6–10 weeks of gestation. The fetal testis releases testosterone, which is converted in the brain to oestradiol. This hormone permanently alters neuronal organization in specific brain areas, for example, the splenium of the corpus callosum. This may

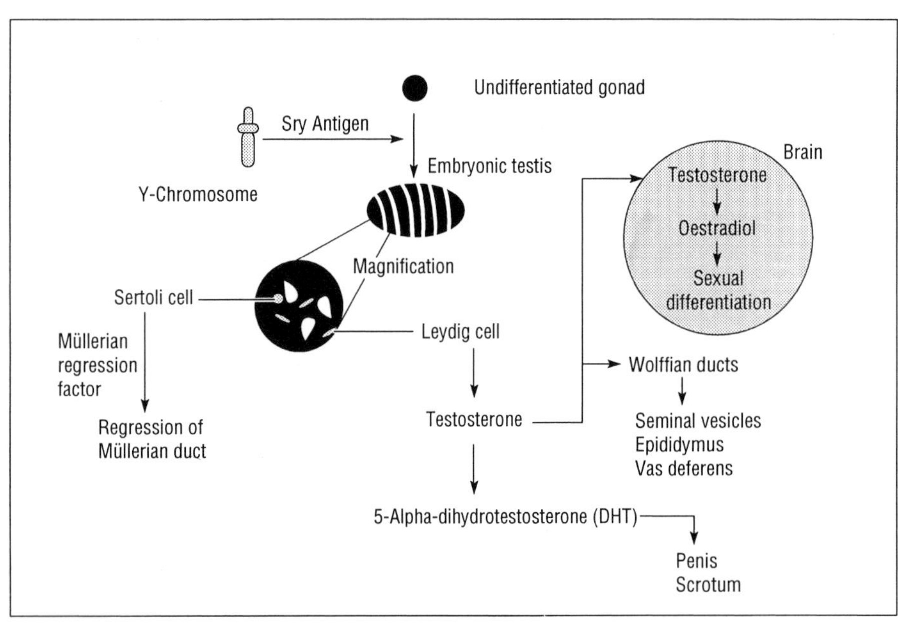

Fig. 19.2 Sexual differentiation of the male.

result in sexual differentiation of sexual and other behaviour in the adult. In rodents, sexual differentiation of the male brain manifests itself in mounting behaviour, and in the absence of the cyclical release of gonadotrophins in the male. In humans, it appears that perception of gender is determined not only by hormones but also by the social milieu.

Puberty: male. After birth, the gonads fall quiescent for some years, until for an unknown reason luteinizing hormone (LH) starts to rise, initially at night, and then during the day as well. This is followed by a more than twentyfold rise in testosterone secretion from the testes, while germ cells of the seminiferous epithelium mature and, together with their supporting Sertoli cells, begin to produce spermatozoa. This is stimulated by local action of testosterone on the tubules, together with follicle-stimulating hormone (FSH). Testosterone then acts as either a hormone, or as a prohormone, through conversion to DHT to enlarge the larynx, the accessory sex organs and the external genitalia, and to produce the male pattern of body hair.

The testes produce a protein called inhibin, which feeds back to the anterior pituitary gonadotroph to limit FSH release, while testosterone feeds back to the anterior pituitary and probably also the hypothalamus to inhibit LH release. The hormone acts in other parts of the brain to mediate sexual and aggressive behaviour, although little is known about the neuroanatomical and neurophysiological aspects of this function of testosterone.

Puberty: female. The cause of puberty onset in girls, as in boys, is unknown, although there are theories which principally involve a postulated maturing of as yet unidentified brain systems, or alterations in brain sensitivity to the negative-feedback effects of oestrogens. Yet another theory holds that the timing may be dictated by the maturation of ovarian follicles as a function of body growth and weight increase. The follicles secrete oestrogens, which precipitate puberty. It is known that leaner, more athletic girls enter puberty later than those who are heavier. Also, anorexia nervosa, which results in prepubertal female body weights, is associated with anovulation.

For some reason, one follicle takes off, and through a huge proliferation of follicular cells matures to a diameter of around 2 cm. Follicle theca interna cells produce androgens, which pass into the granulosa cells of the follicle, where they are aromatized to oestrogens. At the same time, the ovum undergoes meiotic divisions. About 5 days prior to ovulation, plasma oestrogens rise markedly. This oestrogen 'primes' the anterior pituitary

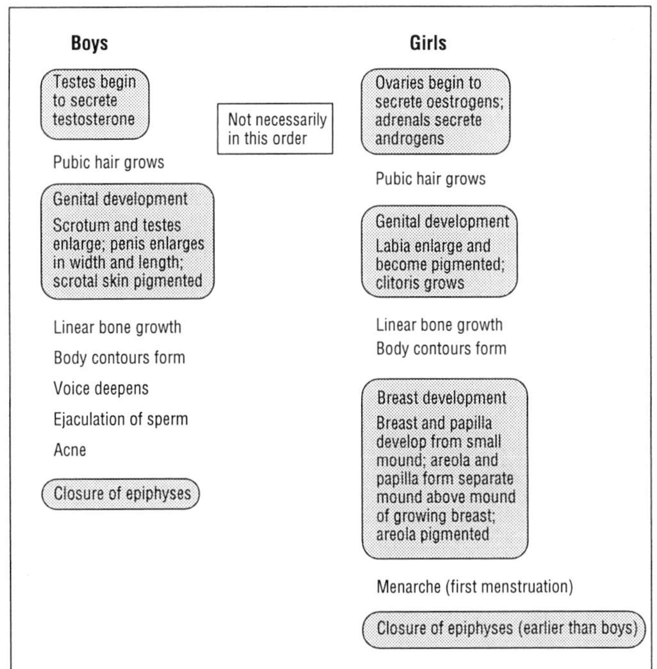

Fig. 19.3 Puberty.

cell, which becomes hypersensitive to the hypothalamic peptide gonadotrophin-releasing hormone (GnRH; see page 66). In humans at least, the net result on the brain is to 'entrain' the system that controls GnRH, so that the neuropeptide is released in 90 minute pulses into the hypothalamic–pituitary portal circulation. This continuous and steady rhythm is needed for fertility. What then follows is the normal menstrual cycle (described in more detail on page 49).

Oestrogen targets sensitive tissues in the body, where it effects its production of the secondary sexual characteristics. Most noticeable is the increase in breast size, and the formation of body contours through the distribution of body fat. (*Note that in males, enough oestrogen is produced to enlarge the breasts, but this is prevented in some unknown way by testosterone.*) As in males, there is a spurt in longitudinal growth (height), although growth stops sooner in girls, due to the closure of the bone ends or epiphyses, which are more sensitive to oestradiol than to testosterone. This explains, to some extent, why women are often shorter than men.

20 Sexual differentiation and development: III

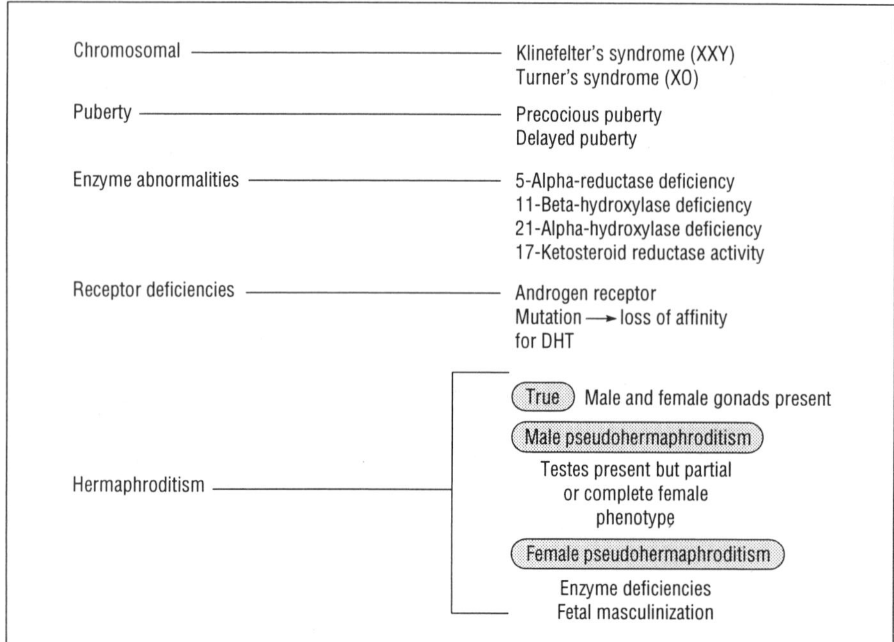

Fig. 20.1 Disorders of sexual differentiation and development.

PATHOPHYSIOLOGY

Although different classifications appear in the scheme shown above, it will become quickly apparent with reading that there is much interdependence and interaction in the occurrence of sexual development disorders. The summary is simply an attempt to provide a quickly grasped and hopefully helpful overview of a complex set of medical problems.

Klinefelter's syndrome. This occurs through the presence of XXY chromosomes. Individuals with this chromosomal set develop hypergonadotrophic hypogonadism. The name implies insufficient secretion of pituitary hormones and consequent deficient gonadal size and function. Although the tissues differentiate normally and a testis develops, the germ cells degenerate shortly after parturition (birth) to leave 'ghost' seminiferous tubules lined with Sertoli cells. The Leydig cells produce abnormally low amounts of testosterone. This results in small testes and high circulating luteinizing hormone (LH), due to a release of the negative-feedback mechanism. These patients may present with gynaecomastia (breast enlargement), azoospermia (complete absence of sperm in the seminal fluid) and with failure of puberty. Treatment is by replacement with androgens, if androgen deficiency is diagnosed.

Turner's syndrome. Here the individual possesses the XO karyotype. The gonads do not develop and the condition is thus also known as gonadal dysgenesis. These individuals are female, short, have a characteristic webbing of the neck and widely spaced nipples, and often present complaining of amenorrhoea (failure to menstruate). They may also show cardiovascular abnormalities, for example, coarctation of the aorta (a congenital narrowing of a short segment of the aorta, which results in hypertension in the upper part of the body).

ENZYME ABNORMALITIES

11-beta- and/or 21-beta-hydroxylase and 17-alpha-hydroxylase deficiencies. These are deficiencies in the enzymes involved in glucocorticoid and androgen production in the adrenal cortex (see page 40). They may be partial or complete, and result from X-linked or autosomal recessive mutations. Deficiencies of 11-beta- and/or 21-beta-hydroxylase result in more 17-hydroxysteroid availability for androgen synthesis (see page 41). This results in virilization of women, with hirsutism (abnormally abundant and distributed body hair), balding and clitoral enlargement. Women born of mothers who suffered from this problem may become masculinized within the uterus. Pregnant mothers with congenital adrenal hyperplasia, where excess androgen production occurs, may also give birth to masculinized daughters.

Such patients also have less of the plasma sex-hormone-binding globulin (SHBG), and the free and therefore physiologically active concentrations of their androgens are abnormally high. Plasma and urinary 17-hydroxysteroid levels are high.

Female patients with congenital adrenal hyperplasia may be treated with low dose prednisolone to reduce ACTH output, and excess androgen may be counteracted with androgen receptor blockers such as cyproterone acetate. Hirsutism is treated also with oestrogen–progestogen combinations. A female with ovaries, that is, exclusively female gonadal structures, but with masculinized genitalia, is termed a female pseudohermaphrodite. Very rarely, some individuals possess both testes and gonads, and are termed true hermaphrodites.

Deficiency of 17-alpha-hydroxylase results in failure of androgen production in gonads and adrenals. Failure to produce androgens results in male pseudohermaphroditism, where primary sexual differentiation has failed; puberty is delayed; and although testes are present, the genital ducts, external genitalia and body contours exhibit a female phenotype.

Androgen resistance. Some males have androgen receptors which are mutated, and through a mutation of just one amino acid in the region of the receptor where androgen is normally bound, the receptor does not bind androgen. Occasionally, the receptor is absent altogether. This is called testicular feminization, and results in an XX phenotype which is identical to that of a woman. The external genitalia are female, although the uterus is short and blind-ended. In these individuals, the Wolffian ducts have failed to develop.

5-alpha-reductase deficiency. This is a rare deficiency of the enzyme that converts testosterone to dihydrotestosterone (DHT) in target tissues. Secondary sexual characteristics, such as voice deepening, pubic and axillary (armpit) hair growth, increased muscle mass and phallus enlargement, which result from testosterone action as a hormone in its own right, are normal, but DHT-dependent structures are abnormal. Features include a labia-like scrotum at birth, failure of development of the prostate gland, and the retention of a urethral opening at the base of the penis and just beneath it.

In men, hypogonadism due to any cause results in low or absent testosterone production. These men present with eunuchoidal features, for example, gynaecomastia; distribution of body fat over buttocks and bony prominences of the trunk; abnormal growth of the long bones; absence of normal androgen-dependent muscular development; scanty secondary sexual hair (face, arms, legs, trunk); small scrotum and a voice that did not break. If the hypogonadism was shown to be due to failure of gonadotrophin production at puberty, the condition is termed hypogonadotrophic hypogonadism, whereas if gonadotrophin levels are high (for example in Klinefelter's syndrome), the condition is termed hypergonadotrophic hypogonadism. Raised gonadotrophins are due to failure of negative-feedback through low androgen production.

Depending on the nature of the problem, treatment may be with androgens, or with stimulators of gonadotrophin release, such as GnRH.

21 Female reproduction: I

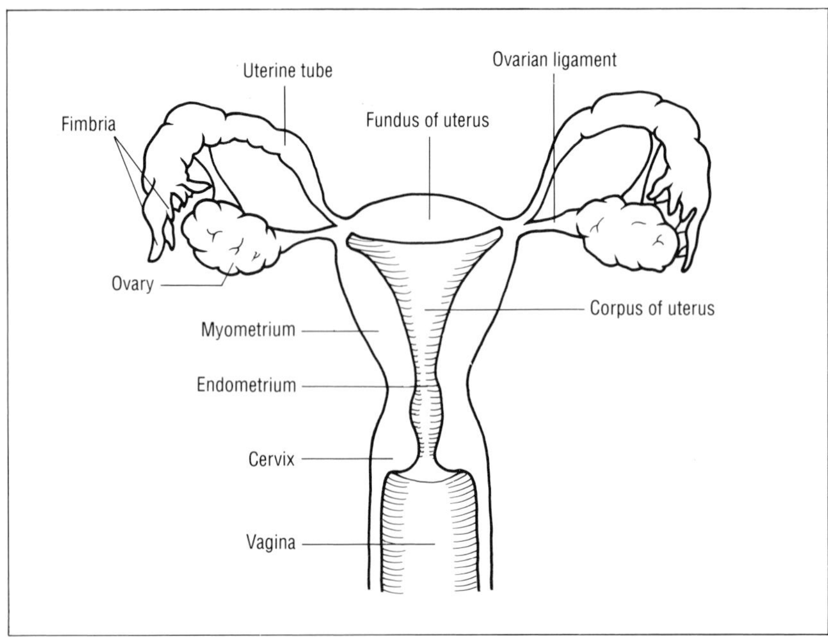

Fig. 21.1 Human female reproductive organs.

FEMALE REPRODUCTIVE ORGANS

The most important female reproductive organs are the ovaries, the ovarian tubes, the uterus and the vagina. The ovaries produce the oestrogens, progesterone and the ovum. After ovulation, the ovum is released into the abdominal cavity, where it is swept up by the fimbriae of the oviducts, and passes into the ovarian tube. Here it may be fertilized, and the fertilized ovum, or morula, passes into the uterus, where it is implanted into the uterine endometrium and grows to become the fetus. Usually, a single ovum is released each cycle from the human ovary.

The menstrual cycle. The principal functions of the female reproductive system are to produce the ovum and to ensure that it is fertilized, nurtured and allowed to grow to term, and to expel it safely into the external environment. The production of the ovum depends upon the orchestration of a number of hormone-dependent events which culminate in ovulation. Inside the ovary during each cycle, many follicles or groups of cells are developing, but only one will develop fully and the others will undergo atresia (degeneration). The follicle develops under the influence of luteinizing hormone (LH), which stimulates oestrogen production, and follicle-stimulating hormone, (FSH) which promotes follicular growth and induces LH receptors. The ovarian granulosa cells produce a protein hormone, inhibin, which is able to suppress FSH secretion from the pituitary. It has been found that subunits of inhibin can actually stimulate the release of FSH, and so the protein may have a complex but important role in the regulation of follicular maturation.

Oestrogen is produced by the ovary during follicular maturation, and stimulates glandular proliferation of the inner lining or endometrium of the uterus: the proliferative phase. At the same time, the hormone stimulates the synthesis of progesterone receptors, thus preparing the uterus for the arrival, later, of large amounts of progesterone. This hormone makes the endometrium secretory, in preparation for the fertilized ovum. The vagina, too, alters cyclically. As oestrogen rises, so the vaginal epithelium proliferates. If fertilization does not occur, then towards the end of the luteal phase (see below) the epithelium is invaded by leukocytes and cast off by the underlying epithelium, representing new growth at the beginning of the next cycle.

The characteristics of the cervical mucus are dependent on the hormonal milieu. During the follicular phase, the mucus is watery, but progesterone changes the mucus to a more viscous form, with minute channels through which the spermatozoa pass on their way to the ovum.

During the pre-ovulatory or follicular phase of the cycle, circulating FSH is high, but as oestrogen and inhibin concentrations rise, they feed back to suppress FSH release. Feedback of oestrogen keeps LH release low as well. Through an as yet unknown mechanism, the rising oestrogen sensitizes the pituitary gonadotrophs to GnRH. Oestrogens may also alter the tonic neurotransmitter influences which control the regular episodic release of GnRH into the portal circulation.

At maturation, the follicle, which is now termed a Graafian follicle, produces less oestrogen and more progesterone, and these hormones appear to act in concert to produce, together

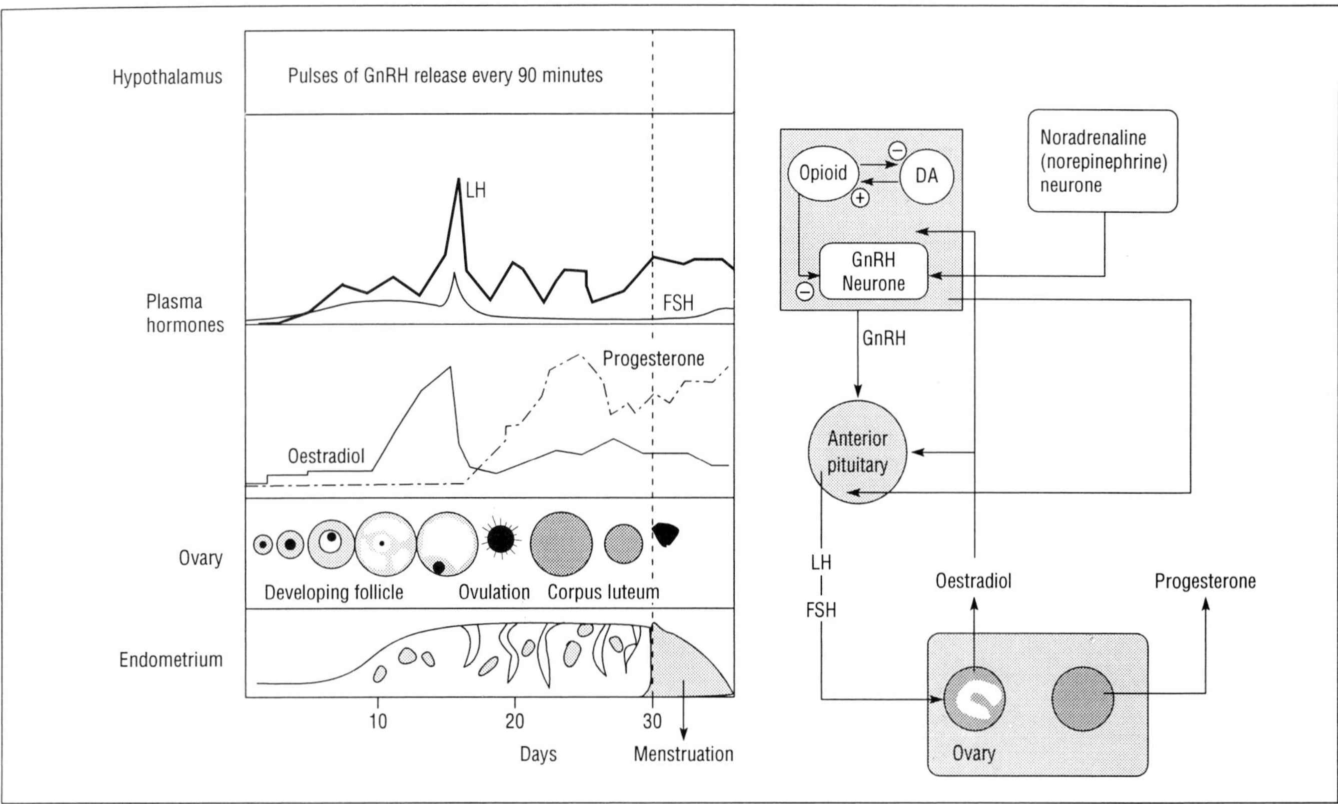

Fig. 21.2 Human menstrual cycle.

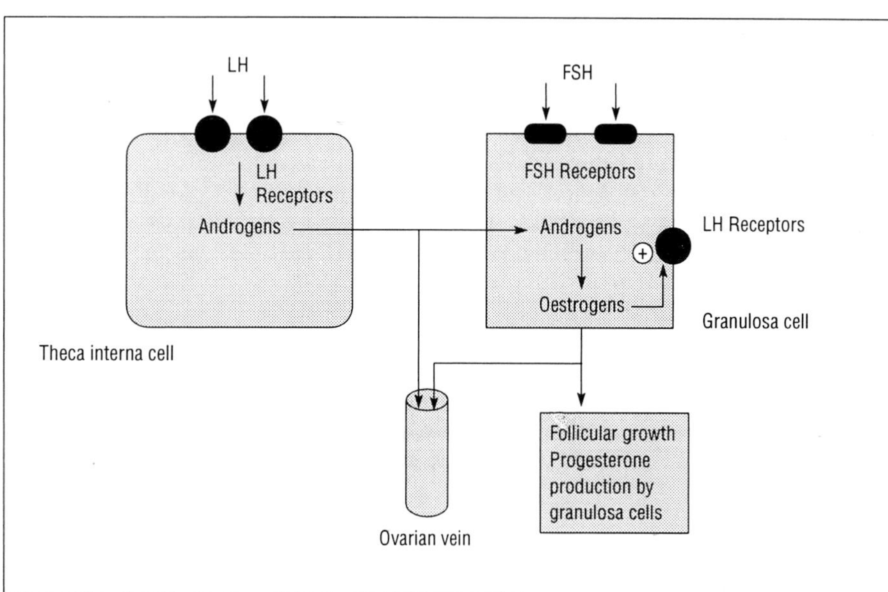

Fig. 21.3 Control of follicular growth by luteinizing hormone and follicle-stimulating hormone.

with the GnRH, a massive release of LH into the bloodstream. The LH causes the follicle to rupture, and the ovum is released. The follicle now becomes the progesterone-secreting corpus luteum (yellow body) and the postovulatory period is termed the luteal phase of the menstrual cycle. If fertilization does not occur, the corpus luteum gradually releases less and less progesterone as it runs its limited lifespan and becomes the corpus albicans (white body). The spiral arteries shrivel; the endometrium collapses due to a lack of blood; and the lining is lost with the menstrual flow. The events described above are termed the menstrual cycle, and occur approximately monthly for the reproductive life of women.

The menstrual cycle varies with the individual, but is taken on average as 28 days, and is numbered from the first day of vaginal bleeding or menses.

22 Female reproduction: II

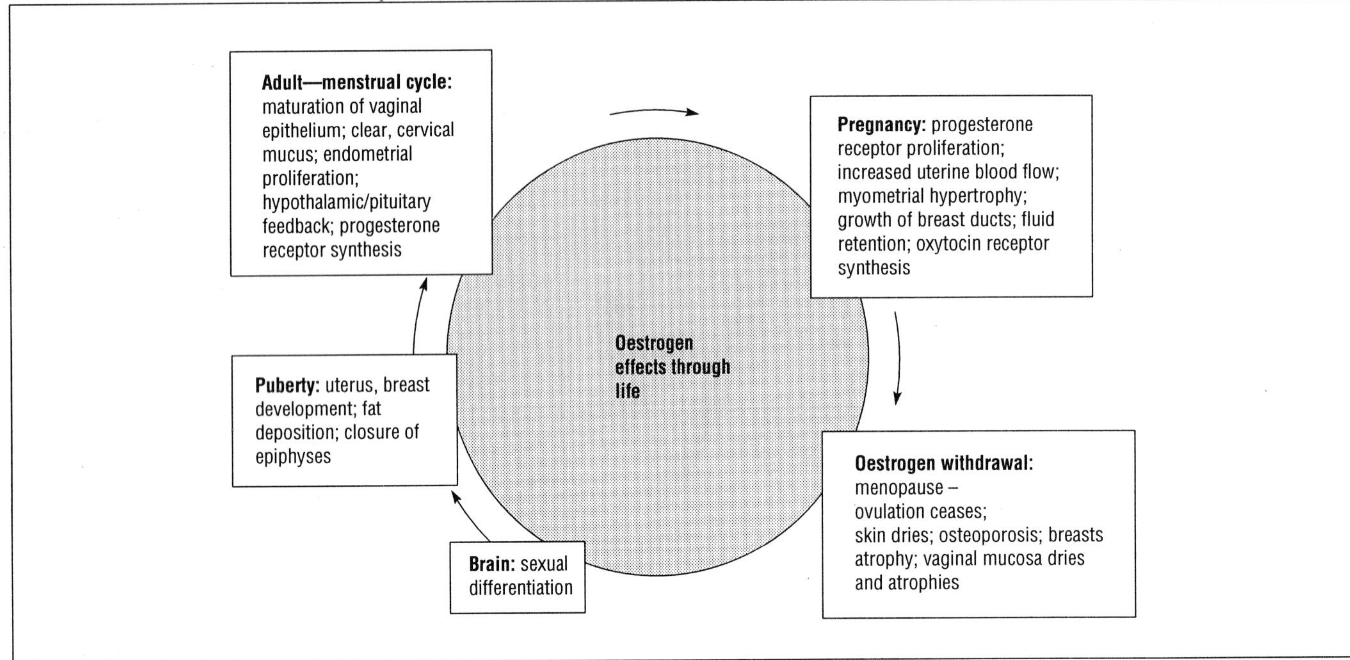

Fig. 22.1 Oestrogen effects.

PHYSIOLOGICAL ACTIONS OF OESTROGENS

The effects of the oestrogens can be classified in chronological order of the major reproductive events of the female. Overall, their main influence is on the maintenance of fertility.

Sexual differentiation. During fetal development, oestrogens are not required for the normal differentiation and development of the female genitalia and accessory sex organs, but they are needed for sexual differentiation of the brain (see also page 44). During the first trimester of pregnancy in the human, the hypothalamus and several other parts of the brain become structurally and possibly functionally differentiated with respect to female behaviour, and the male brain is masculinized by oestrogen, formed locally in the brain from androgen of fetal testicular origin.

Puberty. The cause of puberty onset in humans is unknown (see page 45), but may be due to altered brain sensitivity to oestrogens, allowing the onset of 'positive-feedback' of oestrogens in the hypothalamus, which results in the first ovulation. During puberty, oestrogens stimulate development of breast stroma and ducts, and of the uterus endometrium, myometrium and vagina. The oestrogens cause the pigmentation of the nipples and of the external genitalia, and they stimulate the closure of the epiphyses, the ends of the long bones. The epiphyses are more sensitive to oestrogens than they are to androgens, which is one reason why women are generally shorter than men. Oestrogens cause fat deposition in the tissues, which results in the characteristic contours of the human female.

Adult. In the adult female, oestrogens maintain the menstrual cycle and female sexual behaviour. In humans, much behaviour is learned, and it is difficult to determine to what extent sexual behaviour is oestrogen-dependent or maintained through learning. There is little doubt, however, that in very many species, sexual behaviour is absolutely dependent on the presence of sex hormones. Oestrogens make possible the actions of the hormone progesterone, by stimulating the synthesis of progesterone receptors, notably in the brain and uterus.

Pregnancy. During pregnancy, oestrogens increase the blood flow to and through the uterus; they cause hypertrophy of the uterine myometrium and stimulate breast ductal proliferation. They enhance fluid retention and stimulate uterine progesterone receptor synthesis. Shortly before parturition (birth), oestrogens stimulate the synthesis of oxytocin receptors in the uterus myometrium. Oxytocin is involved in parturition through its contractile action on the uterus (see page 68).

Metabolic effects. Oestrogen inhibits bone resorption, an action which becomes apparent after the menopause, when oestrogen wanes. Oestrogens decrease bowel motility. They affect liver function by stimulating protein synthesis, including that of sex

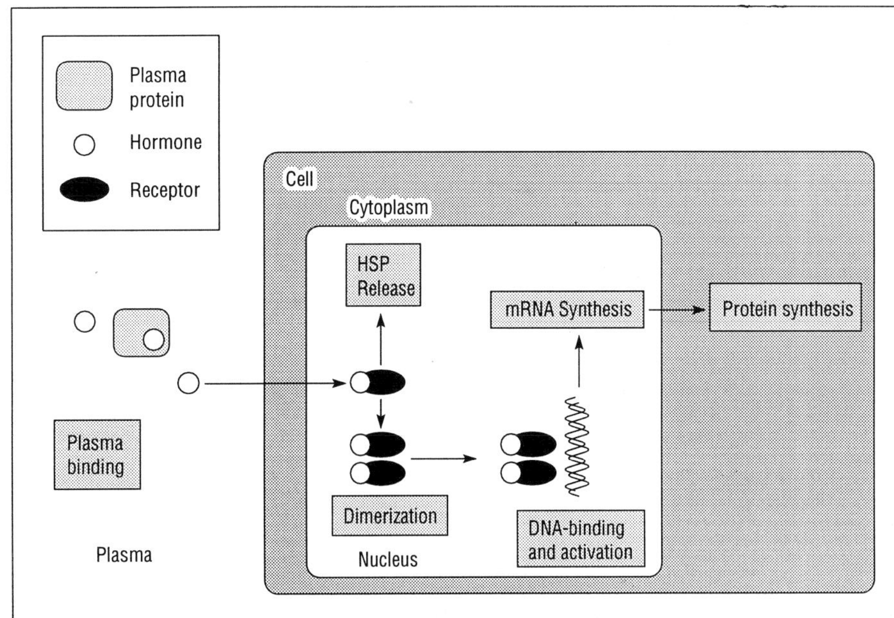

Fig. 22.2 Mechanism of action of oestrogens.

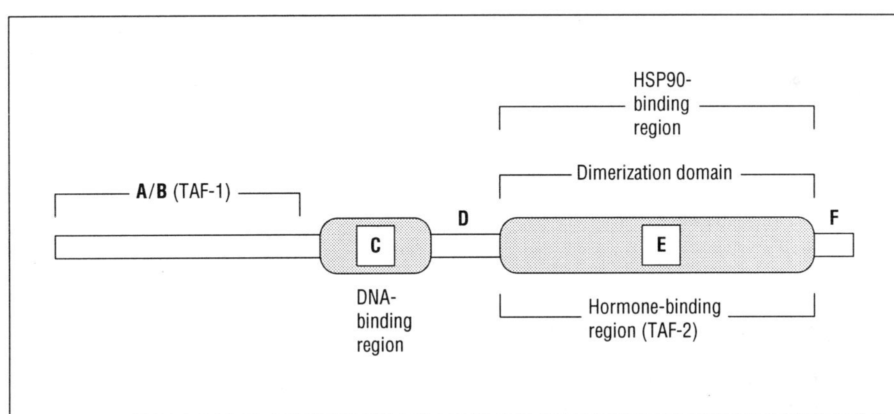

Fig. 22.3 Functional components of the oestrogen receptor.

hormone-binding globulin (SHBG), and of the thyroxin-binding globulin (see page 25).

Oestrogens have important effects on the blood. They increase the chances of coagulation by stimulating the production of factors II, VII, IX, and X; they decrease platelet aggregation; they increase blood levels of high-density-lipoproteins (HDL), and decrease those of low-density-lipoproteins (LDL); LDL is considered a contributory factor in thromboembolic diseases. Oestrogens decrease plasma cholesterol.

Menopause marks the cessation of natural female reproductive life. The ovaries no longer produce ova, and the secretion of oestrogens declines and eventually ceases. As a result, the skin becomes inelastic and withered. The breasts and vagina atrophy, and the latter becomes dry and irritable through the cessation of mucus secretion. Bone resorption occurs, with the attendant danger of fractures.

The symptoms of menopause can be prevented and kept at bay through the use of hormone replacement therapy (HRT; see page 59). In addition, it is now possible for a postmenopausal woman to have children through the use of artificial insemination and surgical implantation of a fertilized ovum.

MECHANISM OF ACTION OF OESTROGENS

Oestrogens travel in the bloodstream, largely bound to plasma proteins, and diffuse into the cell and the nucleus where they bind to specific receptor proteins. As a result of hormone binding, the receptor dissociates from a heat shock protein with which it is associated (see also page 16); two molecules of the receptor dimerize and bind to the DNA at specific hormone response elements (HRE), then initiate transcription and subsequent protein synthesis.

The oestrogen receptor protein has been characterized, and has different multifunctional domains, some of which are still being worked out. The receptor has at least two transcriptional activation functional sites (TAF-1 and 2), a DNA-binding domain, which is similar for many of the DNA-binding receptors, and a hormone-specific binding domain. Sites of dimerization and where the heat shock protein (HSP90) binds, have also been described.

23 Female reproduction: III

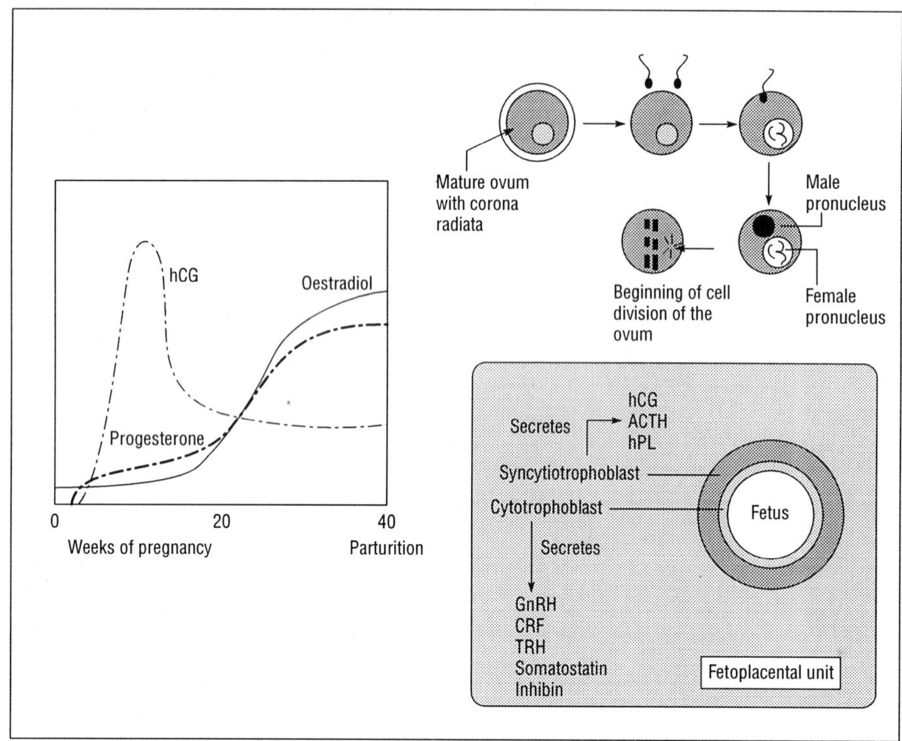

Fig. 23.1 Pregnancy.

PREGNANCY

Fertilization and implantation. If a sperm reaches the oviduct and penetrates the ovum, the ovum and sperm pronuclei fuse to form the *zygote*, which now has the normal diploid chromosomal number. The zygote divides mitotically as it travels along the uterine tube, and at about 3 days after fertilization enters the uterus, when it is now termed a *morula*. The cells of the morula continue to divide to form a hollow sphere, the *early blastocyst*, consisting of a single layer of *trophoblast* cells and the *embryoblast*, an inner core of cells which will form the embryo. The trophoblast, after implantation, will form the vascular interface with the maternal circulation. After around 2 days in the uterus, the blastocyst is accepted by the endometrial epithelium, in a poorly understood process that may involve the transmission of hormones from the blastocyst to the host tissues, thus suppressing the normal immune-mediated rejection response. Oestrogens and progesterone may be important in the process of implantation. This embedding or implantation process triggers the 'decidual response', involving an expansion of a space, the decidua, to accommodate the embryo as it grows. The invasive trophoblast proliferates into a protoplasmic cell mass called a *syncitiotrophoblast*, which will eventually form the uteroplacental circulation. By about 10 days, the embryo, or conceptus, as it is often called, is completely embedded in the endometrium.

If the ovum is fertilized and becomes implanted, the corpus luteum does not regress, but continues to secrete progesterone, and within 10–12 days after ovulation the syncitiotrophoblast begins to secrete a protein hormone, *human chorionic gonadotrophin (hCG)* into the intervillous space. Most pregnancy tests are based on the detection of hCG, which takes over the role of luteinizing hormone (LH) and stimulates the production of progesterone, 17-hydroxyprogesterone and oestradiol by the corpus luteum. It is likely that the same corpus luteum receptors that bind to LH also recognize and respond to hCG. Both hormones have similar beta-subunit structures, and both produce identical biological responses through the activation of the G protein/adenylate cyclase/cAMP system. Together with another hormone, *inhibin* (see page 45), hCG may also serve to inhibit gonadotrophin secretion by the anterior pituitary. It may also

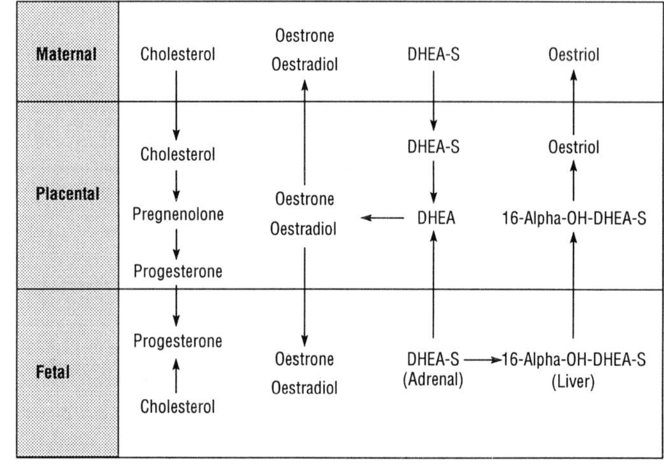

Fig. 23.2 Oestriol biosynthesis.

act as a trophin in the fetus, stimulating production and secretion of steroid hormones involved in, for example, sexual differentiation of sex organs and the brain during the first trimester of pregnancy. Plasma levels of hCG reach a peak between the ninth and fourteenth week of pregnancy, when luteal function begins to fade, and by 20 weeks, both luteal function and plasma hCG have declined.

The syncitiotrophoblast secretes another hormone, *human placental lactogen (hPL)*, whose plasma levels in the maternal circulation (but not in that of the fetus) rise concomitantly with placental growth. Its function may be to inhibit maternal growth hormone production, and it has several metabolic effects, notably being glucose-sparing and lipolytic, possibly through its anti-insulin effects. As a result, the placenta ensures a plentiful supply of glucose, free fatty acids and amino acids for the fetus.

The corpus luteum synthesizes another hormone, *relaxin*, which relaxes the uterine muscle. The hormone is detected in the ovarian venous drainage, is present throughout pregnancy, rises in late gestation, but is rarely found in the plasma of non-pregnant women. Relaxin targets the pubic symphesis, that is, the point of fusion of the pubes, and softens this by converting the connective tissues from a hard to a more fluid consistency. This will facilitate the widening of the pubis to allow the fetus to pass through. Relaxin achieves this effect by increasing the secretion of two enzymes, collagenase and plasminogen activator, both of which dissolve collagen. In late pregnancy, relaxin may be synthesized by the myometrium, the decidua (the mucous membrane which lines the pregnant uterus) and by the placenta.

The placenta, which takes over from the corpus luteum the production of the hormones of pregnancy, is part of what is termed the fetoplacental unit. The placenta attains its mature structure by the end of the first trimester of pregnancy. Its functional unit is the chorionic villus, consisting of a central core of loose connective tissue, packed with capillaries which communicate with the fetal circulation. Around the core are two layers of trophoblast, an inner layer of cytotrophoblast cells and an outer syncytium. The placenta is not only an endocrine organ, but it provides nutrients for the developing fetus and removes its waste products. The fetoplacental unit produces many of the hormones released by the hypothalamic–pituitary–gonadal axis.

Steroidogenesis. Cholesterol is supplied by the maternal circulation, and undergoes side-chain cleavage in the syncitiotrophoblast to form *progesterone*. Progesterone concentrations rise progressively during pregnancy, and a major function of the hormone is thought to be its action, together with relaxin, to inhibit uterine motility, partly by decreasing its sensitivity to oxytocin. The placenta lacks 17-hydroxylase and therefore cannot produce androgens. This is done by the fetal adrenal, and the androgens thus formed are the precursors of the oestrogens. The placenta converts maternal and fetal dehydroepiandrosterone sulphate (DHEA-S) to testosterone and androstenedione, which are aromatized to oestrone and oestradiol.

Another enzyme lacking in the placenta is 16-hydroxylase, so the placenta cannot form oestriol and needs DHEA-S as substrate. Oestriol passes into the maternal circulation, where it is conjugated in the liver to form the more soluble oestriol glucuronides, which are excreted in the urine, and levels of oestriol are used as an index of normal fetal development. If the fetus lacks a pituitary gland, no ACTH is produced and no DHEA-S, and therefore no oestriol, although oestradiol and oestrone levels are normal. (*Note that although the fetoplacental unit does produce ACTH, not enough is secreted to make up the deficiency*.) This also happens if the placenta lacks sulphatase activity. The consequences of oestriol deficiency are delayed labour and intrauterine death, unless caesarean section is carried out. Such mothers are resistant to oxytocin administration, suggesting a deficiency of oxytocin receptors, which are normally induced at term by oestradiol. Another important role of oestrogens is to stimulate the steady rise in maternal plasma *prolactin*. Prolactin, which is the postpartum lactogenic hormone, may serve in pregnancy to regulate storage and mobilization of fat, and to aid in maintaining metabolic homeostasis during pregnancy.

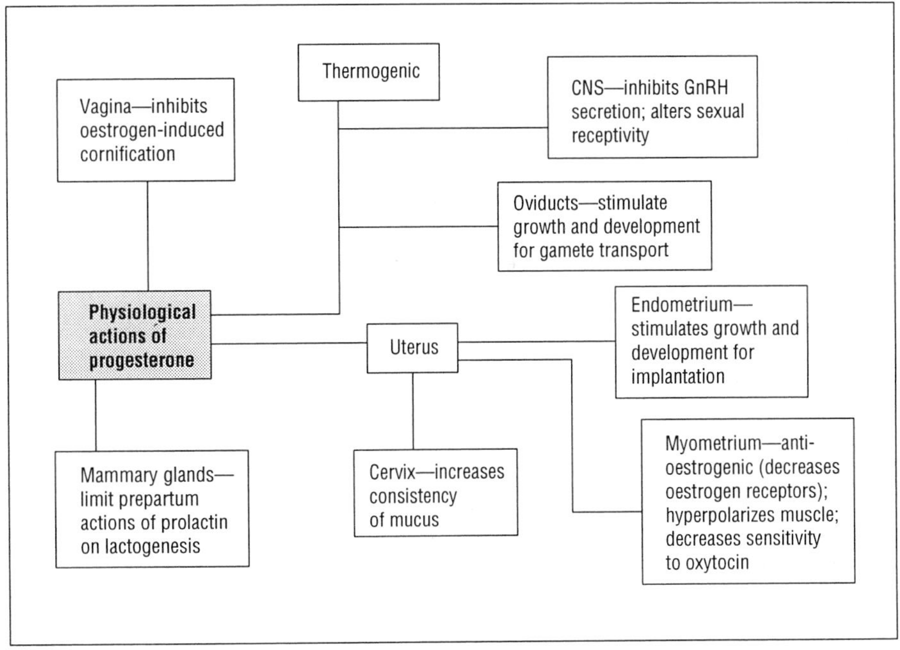

Fig. 23.3 Physiological actions of progesterone.

24 Female reproduction: IV

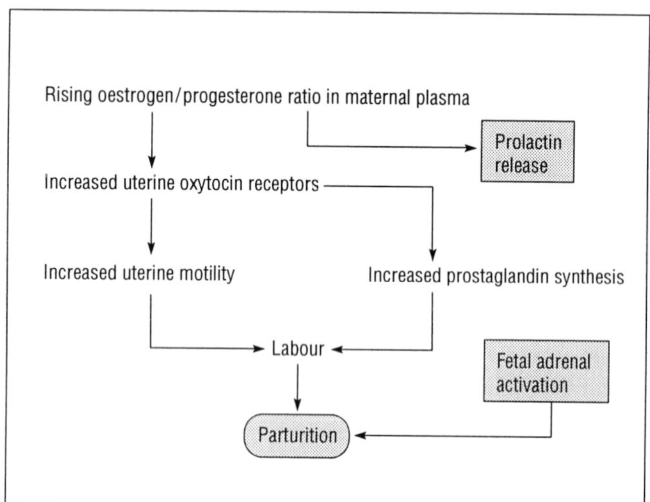

Fig. 24.1 Human parturition.

PARTURITION

The cause of parturition (birth) in humans is unknown, but may be the result of a synchronized set of endocrine-related events. As oestrogen levels rise during pregnancy, they stimulate an increase in uterine oxytocin receptors. The fetus grows rapidly near to the time of birth; its hypothalamus–pituitary system matures and activates the adrenal system, resulting in increased secretion of cortisol; and there is evidence that the fetus produces the oxytocin necessary for the onset of labour.

Cortisol is very important in the initiation of labour in the sheep, but it is not yet known if fetal cortisol plays a similarly pivotal role in human parturition. The distension of the uterus caused by fetal growth may also contribute to increased oxytocin receptor synthesis. Oxytocin, through its receptors, may also stimulate prostaglandin (Pg) synthesis, particularly of $PgF_{2\alpha}$ and PgE_2. The prostaglandins are a group of oxygenated, unsaturated, long-chain fatty acids with profound effects on virtually all tissues, and PgE_2 and $PgF_{2\alpha}$ appear to act through the cAMP second messenger system to increase cytosolic Ca^{2+} and thus uterine contractility. These two have a therapeutic role in the induction of labour. During parturition, there is a profound fall in maternal plasma oestrogen and progesterone concentrations, but it is not known what causes the rapid and sudden changes in the secretion of the female sex hormones during labour.

LACTATION AND THE SUCKLING REFLEX

Although maternal prolactin (PRL) plasma levels rise well before birth, their role in pregnancy is unknown. During pregnancy the breast enlarges, due to the combined effects of PRL, placental lactogen, cortisol, somatotrophin, oestrogens and progesterone on the growth of the mammary lobular–alveolar system, but lactogenesis is virtually absent. Oestrogen and progesterone actually inhibit milk production through a direct inhibitory effect on PRL receptor synthesis.

After birth, however, the concentrations of these two sex hormones are relatively low, and PRL is allowed to play its key role in promoting lactogenesis. Lactogenesis and milk secretion begin very soon after birth. Milk is produced in the cells which line the alveoli, and is composed of lactose (produced from glucose), milk proteins, the most important of which are casein and whey, lipids, divalent cations, and also antibodies, through which the mother transfers certain forms of immunity to the baby. Milk may also transmit some drugs, including drugs of addiction.

There is evidence that PRL stimulates milk production through stimulation of the phospholipase A_2 second messenger system and increased prostaglandin synthesis, resulting in increased mRNA for casein. Cortisol and insulin are essential for this action of PRL. PRL has also been shown to activate the transport of K^+ and Na^+ through an action on the Na^+/Ka^+-ATPase pump, which in mammary tissue is confined mainly to the basolateral membranes of the mammary epithelial cells.

The suckling reflex. PRL secretion from the anterior pituitary lactotroph cell is controlled by a reflex, the neuroendocrine *suckling reflex*. The secretion of prolactin is normally under the inhibitory control of *dopamine* (called prolactin-inhibitory factor, or PIF) from the hypothalamus. The neurotransmitter gamma-aminobutyric acid (GABA) may mediate the release of PIF. When a mother begins nursing, or suckling the baby, the mechanical stimulation of the nipple sends afferent impulses through the anterolateral columns of the spinal cord, some of which converge, eventually, in the supraoptic (SON) and paraventricular (PVN) nuclei in the hypothalamus. Oxytocin is released from neurosecretory terminals in the posterior pituitary, and travels in the bloodstream to the mammary gland, where it contracts the mammary myoepithelial cells, resulting in an explosive discharge of milk. The same reflex somehow lessens or removes the inhibitory influence of dopamine, resulting in PRL release from the anterior pituitary. PRL secretion may also be controlled in the hypothalamus by an as yet undiscovered PRL-releasing factor. Thyrotrophin-releasing hormone (TRH), vasoinhibitory peptide (VIP) and angiotensin II act in the hypothalamus to stimulate PRL secretion from the anterior pituitary.

Milk production is maintained for as long as nursing is continued. In some poorer societies, a mother may be kept lactating for up to 3 years, during which time she is infertile. During nursing, gonadotrophin secretion from the pituitary is inhibited, and sex hormone production remains low. This results in a form of natural contraception: during lactation it is theoretically impossible for conception to occur. Non-lactating women

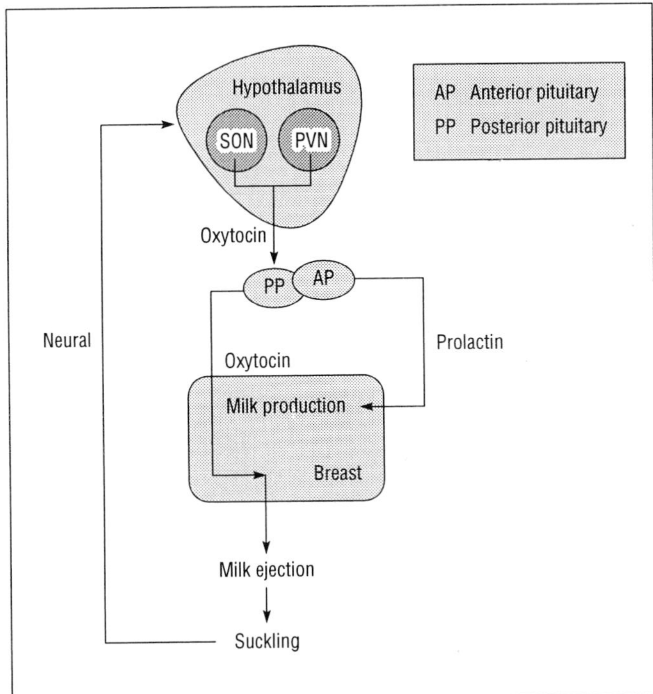

Fig. 24.2 Lactation and the suckling reflex.

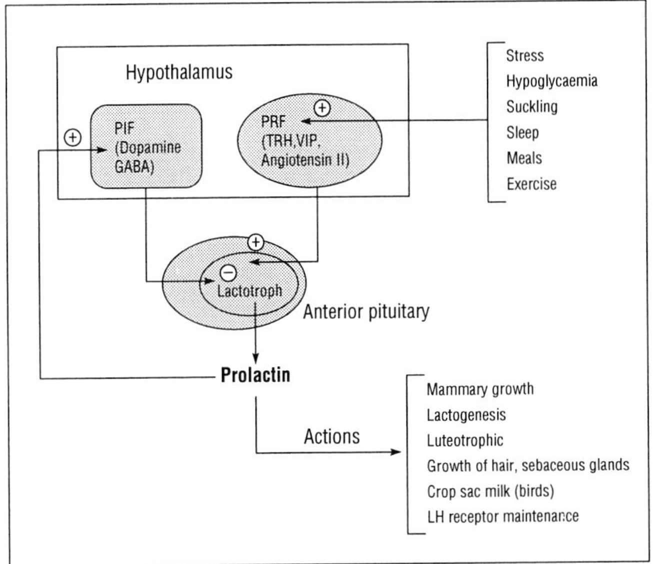

Fig. 24.3 Control of prolactin secretion.

will return to normal cyclic activity within about 4–5 weeks after birth, whereas in lactating women there will be no ovarian follicular development while plasma PRL levels remain elevated. After weaning, or the cessation of suckling, the secretion of oestradiol and of LH increases, reflecting the resumption of normal ovarian function.

Prolactin has many other actions in both males and females, many of which are still poorly understood. It is released in stress, sleep, during eating and exercise, and is involved in hair growth and in the production of crop sac milk in birds. During the normal menstrual cycle it appears to maintain LH receptor production, and also to maintain LH receptors during pregnancy.

25 Female reproduction: V

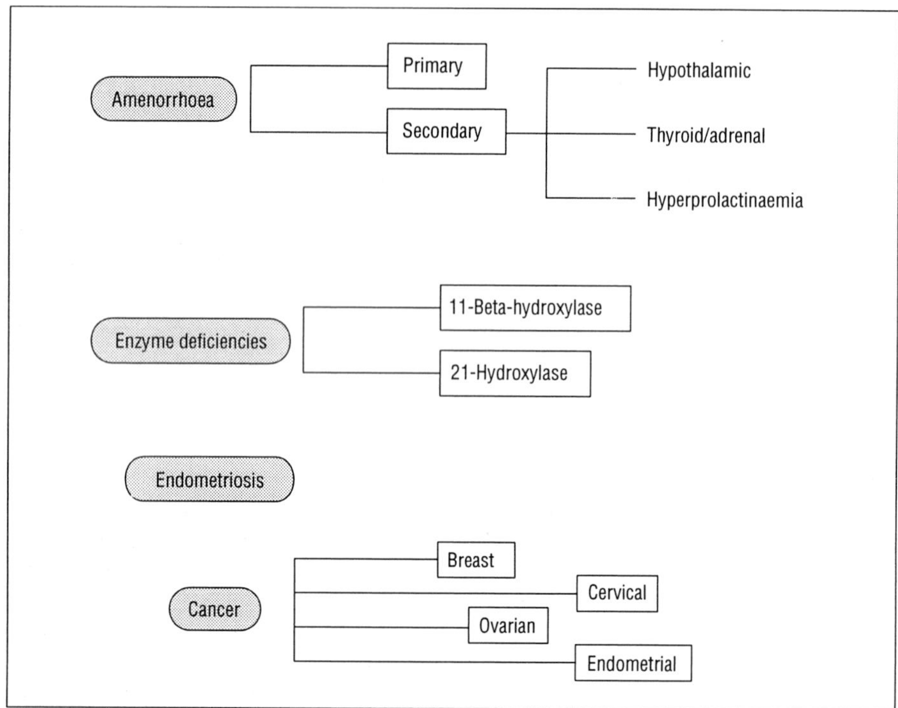

Fig. 25.1 Female reproductive pathophysiology.

FEMALE REPRODUCTIVE PATHOPHYSIOLOGY

Primary amenorrhoea is the failure of menstruation to appear at puberty. Treatment is with gonadotrophin-releasing hormone (GnRH) and sometimes oestrogens.

Secondary amenorrhoea is the stopping of already established menstrual periods. There are several causes.

1 *Hypothalamic disorders*. Amenorrhoea of hypothalamic origin may be psychogenic. Pseudocyesis (phantom pregnancy) is amenorrhoea associated with increased secretion of luteinizing hormone (LH) and prolactin sufficient to maintain a corpus luteum and lactation. It can be cured simply by explaining the condition to the patient.

Anorexia nervosa. Failure to menstruate is associated with prepubertal body weight and low gonadotrophin secretion, similar to that measured in children. It is accompanied by other endocrine disorders of central origin, for example, hypersecretion of cortisol during the 24-hour period, although the normal rhythms of secretion are maintained, and low plasma concentrations of tri-oiodothyronine (T_3), which are similar to those measured in cases of starvation. Regaining adult body weight restores menstruation.

Exercise amenorrhoea may be observed in female athletes whose menstrual cycles are disturbed, perhaps due to loss of body weight. It is known that long distance running or frequent jogging causes the release of brain opioids, which may act directly on GnRH neurones to suppress the episodic release.

2 *Thyroid and adrenal dysfunction*. Hypothyroidism and hyperthyroidism may result in amenorrhoea by altering the production of plasma sex-hormone-binding globulin, and by altering the metabolism of androgens and oestrogens. Women with Cushing's syndrome (see page 40) often suffer from amenorrhoea or oligomenorrhoea (irregular menstruation). The problem may be due to increased brain corticotrophin-releasing factor (CRF) and 5-hydroxytryptamine (5HT) production. CRF has been shown to suppress the production of GnRH, and 5HT inhibits LH secretion from the anterior pituitary.

3 *Hyperprolactinaemia* is frequently associated with amenorrhoea. Hyperprolactinaemia may be due to prolactin-secreting tumours, or to deficient hypothalamic secretion of dopamine, the prolactin-inhibitory factor (see page 55), into the pituitary portal system, and thus to the anterior pituitary. The system is self-perpetuating, since prolactin in turn stimulates the hypothalamic opioid system, which suppresses GnRH production. Treatment is with dopamine receptor agonists, such as *bromocriptine*, to restore menstruation and fertility, or through surgery, to remove the tumour, if present.

Polycystic ovarian syndrome (also called polycystic ovary disease or Stein–Leventhal disease) is the failure of ovarian development and ovulation due to inadequate FSH secretion, resulting in enlarged, distended ovaries which overproduce oestrone and androgens, resulting in hirsutism. The excess oestrone stimulates LH but not follicle-stimulating hormone (FSH) secretion, and follicles do not develop. Treatment is with *clomiphene citrate*, an oestrogen receptor antagonist which blocks the negative-feedback on FSH secretion. *Dexamethasone* may also be given to suppress adrenal androgen production. Purified FSH is also successfully used.

Enzyme deficiencies. 11-Beta-hydroxylase deficiency (see also page 46) results in the hypersecretion of adrenocorticotrophic hormone (ACTH) and adrenal androgens, resulting in hirsutism, amenorrhoea, acne and virilization of external genitalia. Late onset 21-hydroxylase deficiency may cause hirsutism and is treated with dexamethasone to suppress ACTH production.

Endometriosis is the presence of endometrial tissue at ectopic sites in the pelvis. The tissue may penetrate the myometrium, the ovary, the cervix, vagina and the uterine tubes. The ectopic endometrial tissue undergoes the same periodic changes as uterine endometrium, including menstrual bleeding, and may cause severe pelvic pain and dysmenorrhoea (painful menstrual bleeding). The tissue is removed surgically.

CANCER

Breast cancer is the commonest form of cancer in women, and tends to be familial. A woman whose mother and sister have contracted cancer has 4.6 times the chance of contracting breast cancer than a woman without this family history. The disease is exacerbated by oestrogens, and in the past mastectomy (breast removal alone, or together with the lymph nodes of the armpits) was performed, together with the removal of all oestrogen-producing glands. The disease can occur both pre- or postmenopausally, and when breast cancer is diagnosed, the cancer is ablated by surgery and tested for the presence or absence of oestrogen receptors. If it is oestrogen receptor-positive ($ER^{(+)}$), there is evidence that the cancer may respond better to chemotherapy with anti-oestrogens which block the binding of oestrogens to their receptors. $ER^{(+)}$ cancer is treated with *tamoxifen*, an anti-oestrogen, and recent results of extensive tamoxifen trials suggest that both pre- and postmenopausal women survived significantly longer after treatment if their cancers were $ER^{(+)}$. Premenopausal women with $ER^{(-)}$ tumours experienced no benefit from the treatment. $ER^{(-)}$ cancer is treated with other cytotoxic drugs.

Tamoxifen is a partial agonist; it does have some oestrogenic properties, and newer, pure anti-oestrogens are now being used in clinical trials. Another, newer approach is the use of the progesterone receptor antagonist *RU486*. There is evidence that some cancers may actually develop progesterone receptors, and thus become targets for this form of treatment.

Endometrial cancer can be induced experimentally in animals administered with oestrogens, and oestrogens are known to exacerbate (worsen) breast cancer in women, who may also develop cancers in the ovary, cervix or endometrium. Endometrial cancer has been treated successfully with synthetic progestational agents such as *medroxyprogesterone acetate*, and oestrogen-containing oral contraceptives (see page 58) are contraindicated, although the evidence that these actually cause endometrial cancer is not firm.

Ovarian cancer accounts for about 4% of cancers, and about 6% of cancer-related deaths, and this mortality rate is higher than that for endometrial and cervical cancer combined. Treatment is by surgery, followed by the use of a non-hormonally based chemotherapy, usually the antineoplastic agent *cisplatin*. The prognosis is poor, since only 5–15% of patients with the disease in an advanced stage survive longer than 5 years after diagnosis and treatment. It has been suggested that progesterone receptor-positive tumours are an indication of a better prognosis, since they are more likely to respond to progestagens. Ovarian cancer is diagnosed most commonly in postmenopausal women, whose gonadotrophin levels are high due to the lack of sufficient oestrogens to maintain a negative-feedback on the pituitary and hypothalamus. From epidemiological studies, it appears that women who develop breast cancer have twice the risk of subsequent ovarian cancer development than those who do not have breast cancer. Treatment is with non-steroidal cytotoxic drugs, or with progestational agents alone, or together with oestrogens or anti-oestrogens. It has recently been reported that *taxol*, a derivative of the yew tree, may cause regression of ovarian cancers by disrupting the cellular structure of the tumour.

26 Female reproduction: VI

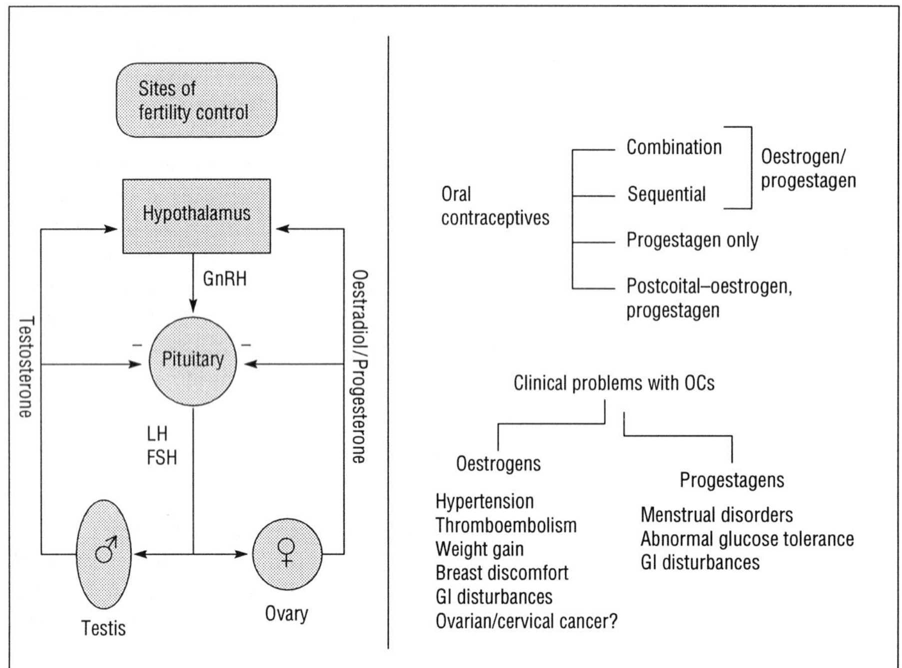

Fig. 26.1 Contraception and fertility control.

Oral contraception is fertility control using orally active synthetic sex hormone derivatives. Oral contraceptives (OCs) represent the most widely used form of oestrogens and progestagens, and constitute the most reliable and effective method for preventing pregnancy in countries where they are widely available.

TYPES OF CONTRACEPTIVE

The first oral contraceptives contained relatively high doses of oestrogen, but with the discovery that high dose oestrogens are associated with endometrial cancer and with cardiovascular accidents, the doses have been greatly reduced.

Combination oral contraceptives contain synthetic oestrogens and progestagens, and examples are given in Table 26.1.

Combination contraceptives act by preventing ovulation through negative-feedback inhibition of gonadotrophin release. This causes minimal follicular development and lower concentrations of endogenously released sex steroids. Women taking combination OCs do not show the early follicular rise of follicle-stimulating hormone (FSH), nor the midcycle rises in FSH and luteinizing hormone (LH). The OC is taken daily for 21 days and withheld for seven, to induce withdrawal bleeding. The OC may also act directly on the uterus and cervix. Cervical mucus becomes more viscous, presumably inhibiting penetration by sperm, and the endometrium does not develop into a suitable matrix for implantation. Missing 1 or 2 days' tablets of OC considerably increases the likelihood of pregnancy, especially since oestrogen doses are relatively low. Combined OC use has been linked with a lower incidence of endometrial and ovarian cancers, and the protective effect reported to last for at least 5 years after cessation of OC use.

Table 26.1 Combination oral contraceptives

Oestrogen	Progestagen
Ethinyloestradiol	Norethindrone
Mestranol	Ethynodiol diacetate
	Laevonorgestrel

Sequential OCs are prescribed so that the user takes oestrogen alone daily for 14–16 days, then oestrogen and progestagen together for 5–6 days, then 7 days without any steroid: this is in order to mimic the natural cycle. Sequential OCs lost popularity in 1976, particularly in the USA, after reports that they were associated with an increased incidence of endometrial cancer.

Some adverse reactions reported after the use of oestrogen-containing OCs are weight gain, especially initially after starting use, menstrual problems, breast discomfort, decreased lactation, hypertension, thromboembolic disorders and endometrial cancer. The possible links between oestrogens in OCs and cardiovascular disease and endometrial cancer are still being intensively studied.

Progestagen only OCs were introduced to eliminate the adverse effects reported with oestrogen use. The progestagen does inhibit FSH and LH release, but a major component of action is due to the thickening of cervical mucus, and endometrial atrophy. The method is not as reliable as oestrogen/progestagen-containing OCs, the success rate being 97–98%, as opposed to 99% for combination OC use. Adverse effects reported with progestagen only OCs are amenorrhoea, changes in plasma high-density-lipoprotein (HDL) and low-density-lipoprotein (LDL); HDL decrease and LDL increase in concentration in plasma; break-through bleeding and 'spotting'; abnormal responses to glucose tolerance tests. Diabetic women have to be monitored carefully if they choose to use these OCs.

Postcoital contraception is the use of large doses of oestrogen alone, or oestrogen in combination with progestagen, within 72 hours of copulation, to block pregnancy. The treatment presumably creates an endometrial environment hostile to the blastocyst. High-dose oestrogens, given in three once-daily doses, can precipitate chemical abortion after implantation has occurred, as they induce withdrawal bleeding after cessation of treatment. This method is associated with dismenorrhoea and occasionally with heavy bleeding, and is not recommended.

A newer, and very controversial agent, *RU486*, has been introduced. This drug blocks the binding of progesterone to its receptor, and can therefore cause abortion by preventing the actions of progesterone in maintaining a quiescent uterus. One dose is given, followed after some days by an injection of prostaglandin $F_{2\alpha}$. This causes uterine contraction and expulsion of the conceptus. The ease with which pregnancy can now be terminated has generated great controversy, particularly in the USA.

OTHER USES OF OESTROGENS

Hormone replacement therapy (HRT) is the use of sex hormones, particularly oestrogens, to replace the lack of endogenous hormones resulting from the cessation of cyclicity of ovarian function. The ovaries are depleted of functional ovarian follicles. The loss of oestrogen is associated with osteoporosis; vasomotor symptoms such as facial 'flushing', particularly during the menopausal period; psychological symptoms; atrophy of the genito-urinary tract; drying of the skin and vaginal discomfort. All these symptoms are ameliorated by oestrogen treatment.

HRT is reported to be associated with a reduction in the risk of cardiovascular disease, particularly coronary artery disease. This may be explained by the fact that after menopause, plasma LDL levels rise and HDL levels fall, and this trend is reversed with HRT. Progestagens in HRT have been reported to increase levels of LDL, and decrease HDL. HRT is administered in the form of sequential daily doses of oestrogen, in a regime similar to that for oral contraception.

OTHER USES OF OESTROGENS AND PROGESTAGENS

Oestrogens have been prescribed for the induction of puberty, to suppress lactation, for osteoporosis, and for treatment of acne in girls. Progestagens are used to stop dysfunctional uterine bleeding, and, controversially, to treat the symptoms of pre-menstrual tension.

27 Male reproduction: I

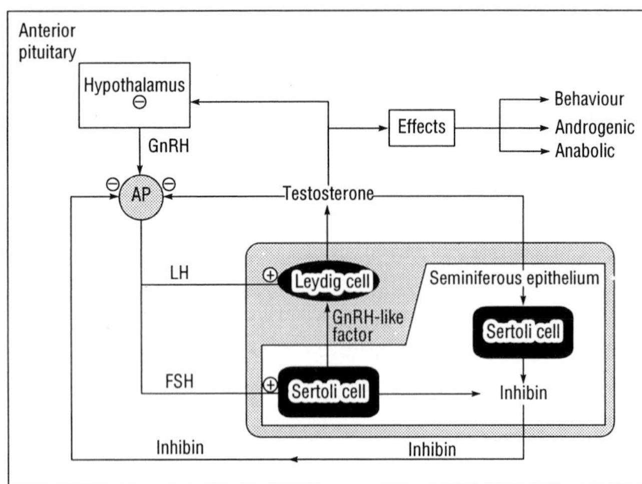

Fig. 27.1 Hormonal control of male reproductive function.

THE TESTIS

The testis is the male gonad, and its primary functions are the production of spermatozoa and testosterone. The spermatozoa are produced in the seminiferous tubules and testosterone is synthesized in the Leydig cell. In the human male, the two testes are in the scrotum, each about 5 cm in length and about 2–3 cm in diameter. The testis is encapsulated within a connective tissue sheath called the tunica albuginea, and consists chiefly of a packed mass of convoluted seminiferous tubules. In each testis, these converge into the rete testis, which opens to feed ductules to the epididymis. The epididymis has a head and a tail, the latter feeding into the vas deferens. It is the vas deferens which is ligated when vasectomy is performed to sterilize a male.

The seminiferous tubules consist of an outer sheath of connective and smooth muscle, surrounding an inner lining containing the Sertoli cells. Embedded within and between the Sertoli cells are the germ cells which produce the spermatozoa, which are released into the lumen of the tubule, and which are stored in the tail of the epididymis. The Leydig cells, also called the intestitial cells, lie between the seminiferous tubules and secrete testosterone.

Control of testis function. The hypothalamus sends episodic pulses (approximately once every 90 minutes) of gonadotrophin-releasing hormone (GnRH) to the anterior pituitary gonadotroph cells, which secrete follicle-stimulating hormone (FSH) and luteinizing hormone (LH). LH targets the Leydig cell, where it stimulates testosterone production through the cAMP second messenger system. FSH targets the Sertoli cell, where it stimulates cAMP and subsequent spermatogenesis, together with testosterone. There is evidence that FSH, perhaps together with *prolactin*, increases the number of receptors on Leydig cells. Another hormone, *inhibin*, is produced by the testis, probably by the Sertoli cell. Inhibin, a polypeptide, is believed to limit FSH release from the pituitary gland by a negative-feedback effect, perhaps on both the pituitary gonadotrophs and directly at the hypothalamic level.

Testosterone biosynthesis in the Leydig cell is from cholesterol, which is converted to pregnenolone. In humans, most of the pregnenolone is 17-hydroxylated and then undergoes side-chain cleavage to yield the 17-ketosteroids, which are converted to testosterone. Once in the blood, approximately 95% of the testosterone is bound to plasma proteins, mainly to a beta-globulin called sex-hormone-binding globulin (SHBG; sometimes called gonadal-steroid-binding globulin, because it also binds oestradiol), and to albumin. Testosterone is metabolized to inactive metabolites chiefly in the liver. These are androsterone and etiocholanolone, which are excreted as soluble glucuronides and sulphates.

Testosterone mechanism of action. The actions of testosterone are complex to unravel, because it acts not only as a hormone in its own right, but also as a *prohormone*. In the target cell, testosterone may be reduced to its 5-alpha-reduced metabolite 5-alpha-dihydrotestosterone (DHT), and also aromatized to oestradiol. In a highly androgen-dependent tissue such as the prostate, testosterone diffuses into the cell, where it is converted to 5-alpha-dihydrotestosterone. This is the active androgen in the prostate gland. DHT binds to an intranuclear androgen receptor which stimulates transcription. The androgen receptor is also able to bind testosterone, and, to a lesser extent, progesterone. In this regard, it is worth mentioning that the androgen receptor exhibits a high structural homology with the receptor for progesterone, although they are distinct receptor types within the larger subfamily of steroid receptors (see page 15). The androgen receptor possesses a hormone-binding domain and a DNA-binding region, consisting of two zinc fingers (see page 14).

Antiandrogens have been synthesized. They compete with DHT for its receptor site. The effective antiandrogens are based on the structure of progesterone, and examples include *cyproterone* and *cyproterone acetate (CA)*, and *flutamide*. In human males, CA causes atrophy of the prostate and seminal vesicles, and a loss of libido. The drug has been used with little success in the treatment of sex offenders. CA will inhibit the progress of acne in teenagers, and the onset of baldness. In women, CA has been used to treat virilization and hirsutism.

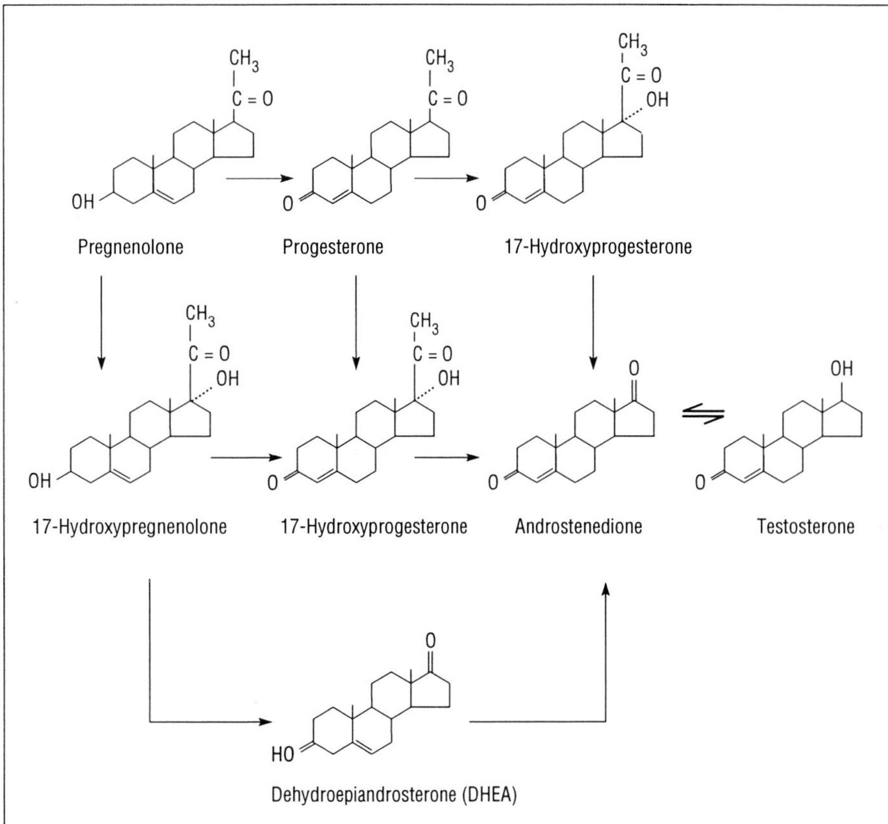

Fig. 27.2 Synthesis of testosterone in testis.

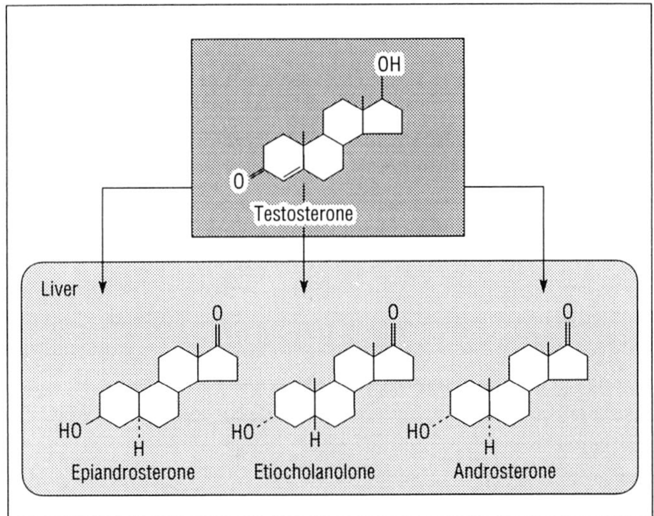

Fig. 27.3 Metabolism of testosterone.

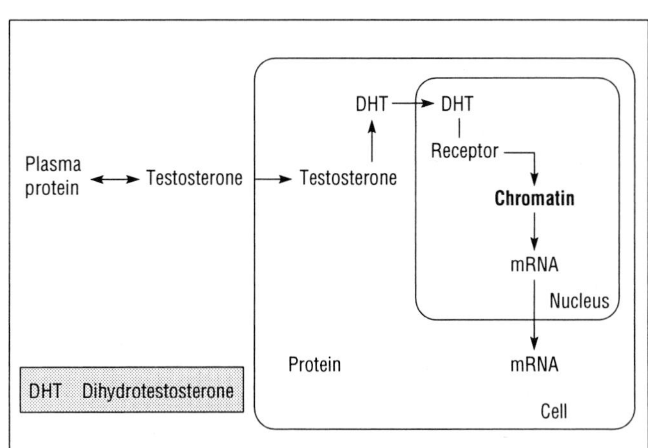

Fig. 27.4 Androgen mechanism of action.

28 Male reproduction: II

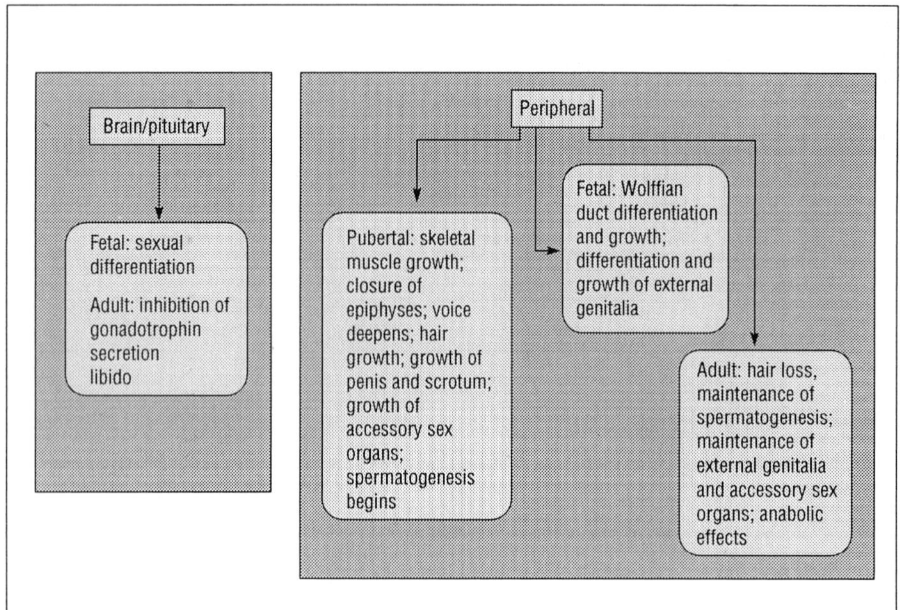

Fig. 28.1 Actions of testosterone.

ACTIONS OF TESTOSTERONE

Actions of testosterone are to establish and maintain the function of the male, as summarized, and to maintain libido in the female. The actions of testosterone can be broadly classified as androgenic ('making maleness') and anabolic (growth-stimulating; creating a positive nitrogen balance).

Brain and spinal cord. In birds and mammals, testosterone sexually differentiates the fetal brain (see page 44). The fetal brain contains androgen and oestrogen receptors, which mediate these actions of testosterone. In fetal rats, testosterone may act to protect neurones from cell death, particularly in the preoptic region of the hypothalamus, in the fifth and sixth lumbar segments of the spinal cord, and in the spinal nucleus of the bulbocavernosus.

In adult rats, the medial preoptic nuclei in the brain are larger than in females, but this difference is eliminated if the males are castrated during the critical period of brain sexual differentiation. Conversely, if neonatal female rats are injected with testosterone, they develop a medial preoptic region similar in size to that of the male. (Gestation in the rat is 21 days, and the critical period for brain sexual differentiation is between Day 18 of gestation and Day 5 postpartum.) Castration of adult rats results in the shrinkage of cell bodies and axons of motoneurones involved in male copulation, and these are restored in size after androgen replacement. Although no evidence is available about these actions of testosterone in humans, there is evidence that testosterone causes changes in the fetal brain during sexual differentiation of the brain at about 6 weeks.

Behaviour. The precise nature of the influence of testosterone on behaviour is unknown, due in part to the limitations of methods of study. In humans, there is no apparent relationship between plasma levels of testosterone and any parameters of sexual or aggressive behaviour. Hypogonadal men display the same competence in producing an erection as do men with normal testosterone secretion. On the other hand, testosterone does stimulate more fantasizing about sex, and in a recent American study, elderly men treated with injections of testosterone reported more sexual fantasizing and a renewed desire to compete in business. It seems that behaviour has a powerful influence on testosterone production, since stress drives it down, as does depression and threatening behaviour from others within a social group. In captive primate colonies, subordinate males have raised prolactin and very much reduced plasma levels of testosterone.

PERIPHERAL ACTIONS OF TESTOSTERONE

A fundamental role of testosterone, together with follicle-stimulating hormone (FSH), is the maintenance of spermatogenesis. It is currently believed that FSH stimulates Sertoli cells to produce cAMP, which stimulates synthesis of a specific protein, androgen-binding protein (ABP), which is secreted into the lumen of the seminiferous tubules. The Sertoli cells also produce the nutrient requirements of the growing and differentiating spermatozoa. Luteinizing hormone (LH) stimulates the Leydig cells to produce testosterone, which binds to ABP, and the complex in some unknown way brings testosterone into close proximity with the developing spermatocytes. ABP may also

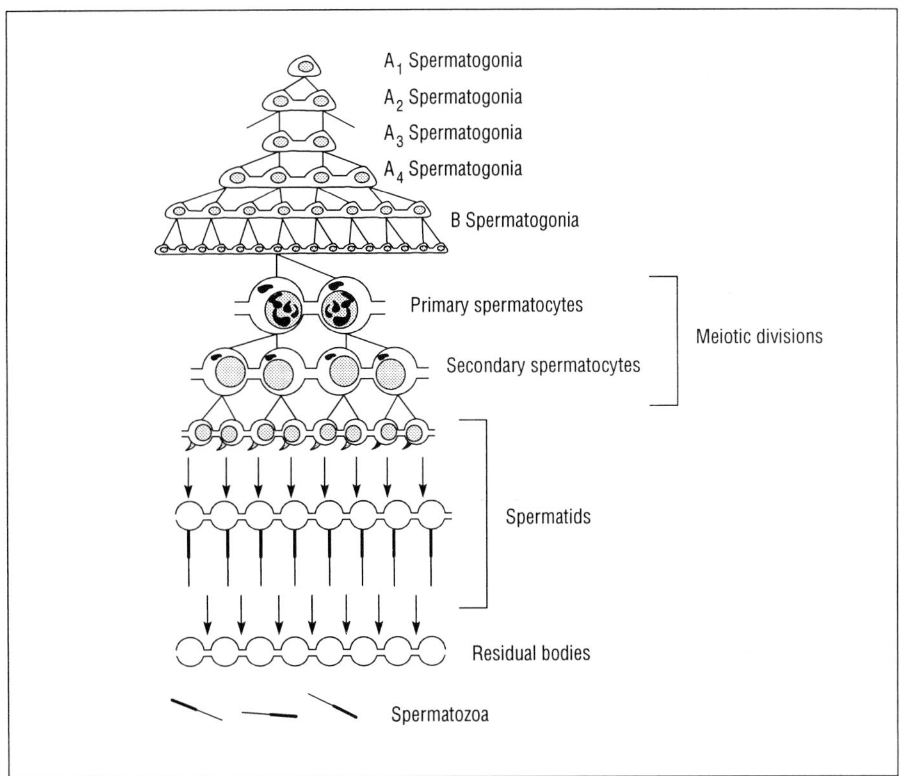

Fig. 28.2 Human spermatogenesis.

function to build up local concentrations of testosterone, and transport the hormone to the epididymis. The Leydig cell also synthesizes oestrogens which bind to ABP, and which are essential for normal spermatogenesis. Growth hormone is essential for early division of the spermatogonia.

About 120 million sperm are produced each day by the young adult human testis. Most are stored in the vas deferens and the ampulla of the vas deferens, where they can remain and retain their fertility for at least 1 month. While stored, they are inactive due to several inhibitory factors, and are activated once in the uterus. In the female reproductive tract, sperm remain alive for 1 or 2 days at most. Sperm remain alive in neutral or mildly alkaline environments, but are rapidly killed in strong acid media. The metabolic activity of sperm increases markedly with increasing temperature, but this also shortens their life considerably.

Accessory sex organs. Testosterone maintains the functions and structural integrity of the *seminal vesicles* and the *prostate gland*. The seminal vesicles are essentially secretory, producing many substances, including large quantities of prostaglandins, fructose and fibrinogen. During ejaculation, the seminal vesicles contract, ejecting their fluid into that carrying the spermatozoa. The fructose is an important nutrient for the sperm, and the prostaglandins aid in the movement of sperm by contracting the uterus and uterine tubes, as well as by reacting with cervical mucus to make it receptive to sperm. During orgasm and emission, the prostate gland secretes a thin, alkaline fluid containing a profibrinolysin, a clotting enzyme, calcium, citrate ions and acidic phosphate. The functions of prostatic fluid are unknown, but they may serve to create a less acidic environment for the sperm and increase their motility.

Anabolic actions of testosterone. Testosterone increases basal metabolic rate through an increase in enzyme and other protein synthesis. Testosterone produces a 10–15% increase in red blood cell production during puberty, and men have about 700 000 more red blood cells per millilitre than women. Testosterone increases muscle mass, despite an apparent absence of androgen receptors in skeletal muscle. The effect may be due to an inhibition of the normal catabolic effects of glucocorticoids in muscle.

29 Male reproduction: III

MALE REPRODUCTIVE PATHOPHYSIOLOGY

Hypogonadism is the failure of the testes to function, that is, to produce testosterone and spermatozoa, and can be due to genetic defects (see page 46). *Primary hypogonadism* refers to abnormalities within the gonad, for example, Leydig cell agenesis (non-development), or failure of Leydig cells in adult life (also called a male climacteric phase). In women, the term 'climacteric' is the time after the last menstruation, and does not imply the pathogenic state that it does in men, since men can retain testis function into old age. Leydig cell failure can occur after mumps. *Secondary hypogonadism* refers to gonadotrophin deficiency or failure to secrete gonadotrophin-releasing hormone (GnRH), and is also called *hypogonadotrophic hypogonadism*.

Hypergonadism means the excess activity of the gonad, which can be *virilizing* due to androgen-secreting Leydig cell tumours, or *feminizing*, due to oestrogen-producing Leydig cell tumours. This is *primary hypergonadism*, whereas that produced through excess GnRH and/or gonadotrophic production is *secondary hypergonadism*.

Androgen resistance is caused by mutations of the androgen receptor, which no longer binds androgen with sufficient affinity for a normal androgenic response to be maintained, or by the complete absence of the androgen receptor.

Gynaecomastia is breast enlargement in males. It usually occurs through abnormal endogenous or exogenous oestrogens. Gynaecomastia accompanied by galactorrhoea (milk production) may be indicative of a prolactin-secreting tumour. Gynaecomastia sometimes occurs in ageing men, which may be because of an increasing oestrogen/androgen ratio in the blood. The condition has also been reported after the smoking of cannabis, which is known to decrease testosterone synthesis and to drive down libido, and, anecdotally, reported to lower ambition.

Impotence is the failure to achieve erection of the penis, and the cause is unknown. Erection is caused by nerve impulses passing through parasympathetic efferents, the nervi erigentes, to the penis. The result is vasodilation of penile arteries, which allows the build-up of arterial blood in the corpus cavernosum and the corpus spongiosum. The corpus cavernosum is one of a pair of cylindrical blood sinuses which form the erectile tissue of the penis or the clitoris, and the corpus spongiosum is a blood sinus surrounding the urethra. These engorge with blood and the penis becomes erect. There is, however, no good evidence that impotence is due to dysfunction of the cholinergic nervous input to the penis. Recently it has been found that erection is associated with the presence of large amounts of the peptide vasoactive intestinal peptide (VIP) in blood of the sinuses, and VIP is present in nerve terminals in the sinuses. Furthermore, VIP produces erections when infused into the sinuses. This discovery may lead to a treatment for impotence. There is much evidence that impotence can be a psychological problem, but it remains to be seen whether psychological disturbances causing impotence are related to reduced release of VIP from nerve terminals in the penis.

Priapism is persistent, painful erection of the penis, and can be produced by drugs such as papaverine. The underlying endocrine basis, if any, of priapism is unknown, and an unrelieved priapism will result, eventually, in fibrosis of the spongy erectile tissue, making future erections impossible to achieve.

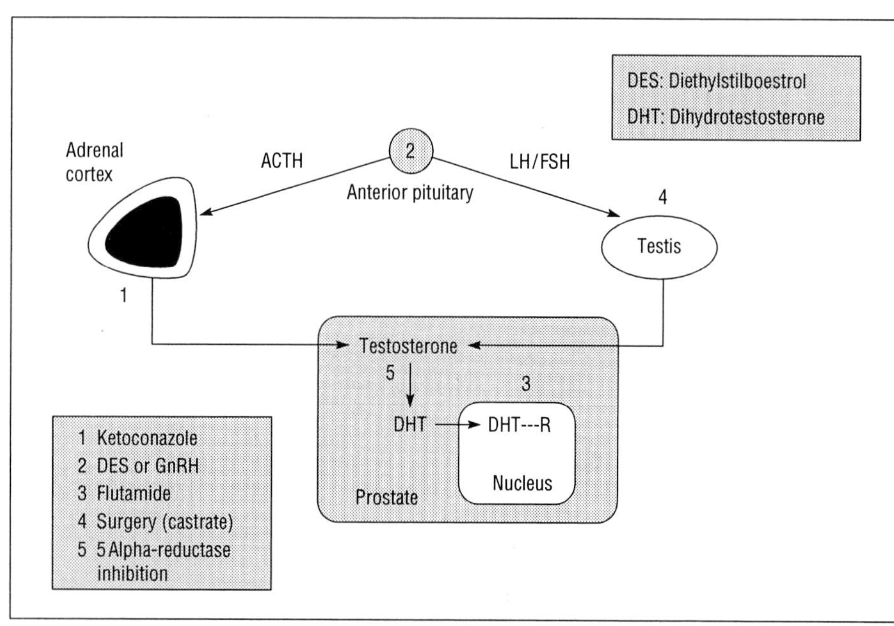

Fig. 29.1 Treatment of prostate cancer.

Prostatic pathophysiology is arguably the most serious part of male reproductive pathophysiology, since it can be life-threatening.

Benign prostatic hyperplasia (BPH) is the growth of the medial lobe of the human prostate, most often in late middle-aged men, until it presses on and begins to occlude the urethra. It is termed 'benign' because it does not invade other tissues and destroy them, or metastasize to distant sites in the body. BPH is androgen-dependent, being strongly stimulated by dihydrotestosterone (DHT), the active androgenic metabolite of testosterone in the prostate gland. The most effective treatment has been the surgical removal of all or part of the gland. The operation can be performed through the bladder (transvesical prostatectomy) or through the urethra (transurethral resection), when prostate tissue is burned away using a heated element. Recently, inhibitors of the enzyme 5-alpha-reductase, which converts testosterone to DHT, have been introduced to treat BPH.

Prostate cancer is carcinoma of the prostate. It is virtually always androgen-dependent, and metastasizes, often painfully, to the spine. When diagnosed in the past, the patient was castrated or treated with large doses of the oestrogen diethylstilboestrol (DES). The aim is to remove the tumour and all sources of androgen production. *Ketoconazole*, a drug used to treat fungal infections, may be prescribed, since it inhibits the synthesis of cholesterol and therefore blocks steroid production in all tissues. A newer and more acceptable treatment is the administration of stable analogues of GnRH, such as *buserelin*. These, if continuously present in the bloodstream, actually shut down anterior pituitary production of gonadotrophins by rendering the gonadotrophs insensitive to GnRH from the hypothalamus. (They do *not* achieve this by down-regulating GnRH receptors.) The result is a chemical castration, which can be reversed by stopping treatment. Another approach is the administration of androgen receptor blockers such as *flutamide*, or *cyproterone*.

When using GnRH analogues, it is advisable when starting treatment to administer the drug together with an anti-androgen. This is because the initial effect of the GnRH analogue is to stimulate a transient increase in testosterone production, which may in turn cause a fatal stimulation of tumour activity.

30 Gonadotrophin-releasing hormone as an example of an endocrine peptide hormone

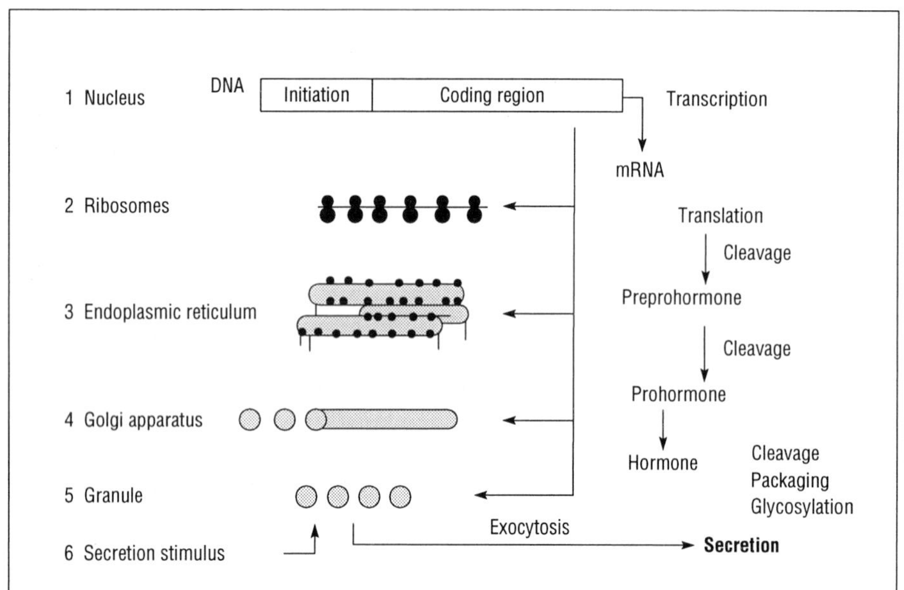

Fig. 30.1 Synthesis and release of peptide hormones.

SYNTHESIS AND RELEASE OF PEPTIDE HORMONES

Peptide and protein hormones are increasing in importance as more and more are discovered, and it is necessary to have at least a basic knowledge of the steps in their synthesis and release. Gonadotrophin-releasing hormone (GnRH), which has been extensively covered in this book, provides an excellent example of a peptide hormone for study, since so much is known about its chemistry, production, release and actions.

Transcription. The first step in the synthesis of a peptide such as GnRH is the transcription of the gene coding for the hormone mRNA. An initiation site on the gene, upstream from the coding region, is activated by a signal from the cytoplasm of the hypothalamic neurone in which it is synthesized. In the case of GnRH, the signal originates from a neurotransmitter, perhaps dopamine, which triggers an increase in cytoplasmic cAMP, resulting in the activation of the gene. Conversely, cAMP production may be inhibited as a result of the action of an opioid neurotransmitter acting on its receptor on the membrane of the GnRH neurone.

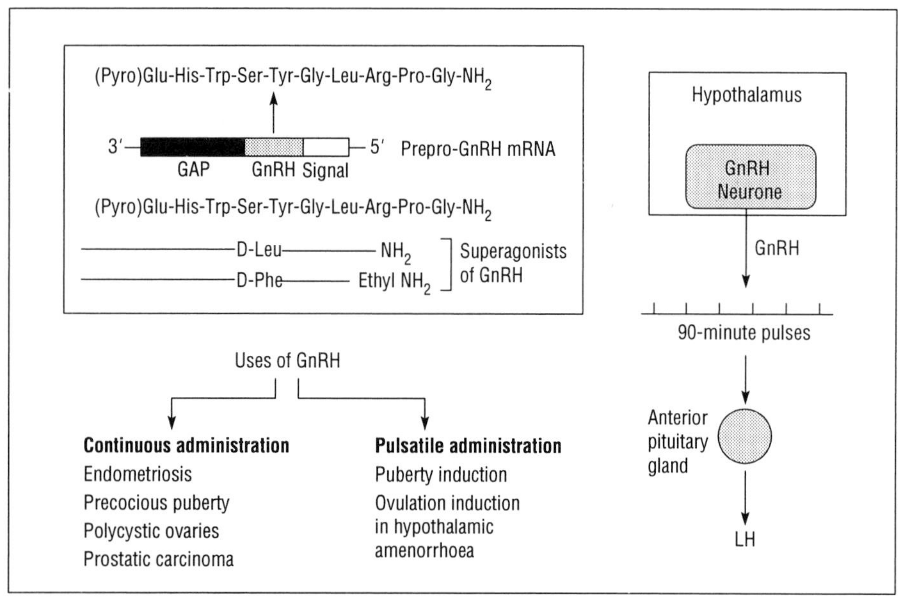

Fig. 30.2 Gonadotrophin-releasing hormone.

Preprohormone. The GnRH mRNA is called prepro-GnRH mRNA, since it will be translated into a large precursor peptide called prepro-GnRH. The mRNA moves out of the nucleus to the cytoplasm, where it is translated by ribosomes on the endoplasmic reticulum into prepro-GnRH. The precursor peptide consists of a signal sequence of 23 amino acids, followed by the sequence of GnRH itself. Following on from GnRH are 56 amino acids, forming the C-terminal portion of the peptide. This latter portion is termed GAP (GnRH-associated peptide), which, incidentally, has been discovered to be an inhibitor of prolactin secretion. This highlights the principle that more than one physiologically active peptide can be generated from a single peptide precursor. The signal peptide sequence at the N-terminal end of prepro-GnRH directs its transfer to the endoplasmic reticulum, and during this processing it is cleaved to form a shorter prohormone.

Cleavage and packaging. From this point, the prohormone is transferred to the Golgi apparatus, where it is cleaved further to from the final hormone, in this case the decapeptide GnRH. The hormone is packaged into storage vesicles and released on demand, in this case the cellular response to neurotransmitter activity. Generally speaking, peptide hormones may be released in response to: the binding of ligands for other receptors on the cell surface; a voltage change on the surface of the cell; a metabolic change within the cell itself.

Exocytosis. The hormone is released from the cell through the process of exocytosis. On stimulation, intracellular free Ca^{2+} and cAMP rise, causing contraction of myofilaments, and the vesicle is guided along microtubules to the cell membrane. The vesicle fuses with the membrane through a process which requires Ca^{2+}. The membrane is lysed and the contents are released into the extracellular space, and enter the bloodstream through neighbouring capillaries. GnRH neurone terminals impinge on the portal vessels, so that on release, a large proportion of exocytozed GnRH enters the portal system.

Structure–function relationships. Once the structure of the hormone is elucidated, attempts are made to synthesize more stable analogues for therapeutic use, and in the case of GnRH, substitution with D-amino acids produces potent analogues resistant to enzyme digestion.

Receptor characterization. The stable analogues are radiolabelled and used to study the localization and properties of the peptide receptor. In the case of GnRH, these are situated on the plasma membrane of the anterior pituitary gonadotroph, and stimulation of the GnRH receptor by GnRH causes a rise in intracellular cAMP paralleled by the secretion of follicle-stimulating hormone (FSH) and luteinizing hormone (LH).

Hormone measurement. Once the hormone has been identified and synthesized in large quantities, antibodies can be raised against the hormone and used to measure it under different physiological and pathological conditions. In the case of GnRH, the availability of a radioimmunoassay enabled the discovery that the hormone is released episodically, approximately every 90 minutes. This episodic release is necessary to maintain gonadotrophin release, and thus fertility, in both the male and the female primate, including humans.

31 Oxytocin

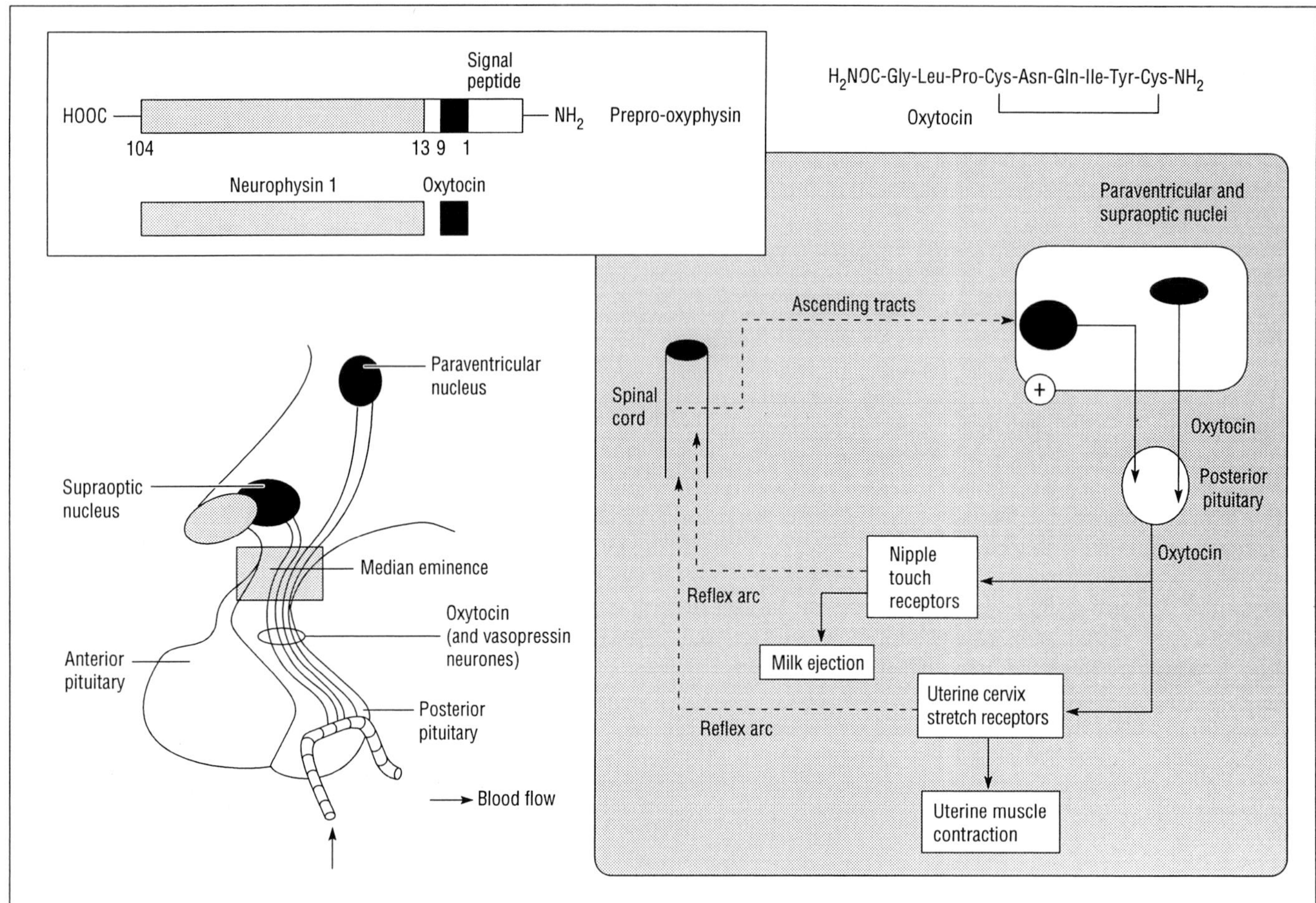

Fig. 31.1 Oxytocin.

BIOSYNTHESIS

Oxytocin is synthesized in the cell bodies of the magnocellular neurones of the paraventricular and supraoptic nuclei of the hypothalamus. Other neurones in the same nuclei produce vasopressin (see page 70). The axons of these neurones pass through the median eminence and terminate in close contact with fenestrated capillaries in the posterior pituitary gland. Both oxytocin and vasopressin are synthesized in the rough endoplasmic reticulum of the cell body, together with proteins called *neurophysins*. Oxytocin and its neurophysin protein (called neurophysin I) are packaged together in the Golgi apparatus in the same vesicle or secretory granule, which also contains the enzymes which cleave oxytocin from the neurophysin as the granules migrate along the axon towards the nerve terminal. It takes about 12 hours for the granule to travel from the cell body to the posterior pituitary. Neurophysin I is occasionally referred to as the oxytocin transport protein. There is evidence that if the neurophysins fail to be synthesized, then oxytocin and vasopressin do not reach the posterior pituitary.

It should be noted that oxytocin neurones send axons not only to the posterior pituitary, but also to higher centres in the brain, where the hormone may serve as a neurotransmitter mediating certain forms of behaviour (see below).

SECRETION

Excitatory cholinergic and inhibitory neurones make synaptic contact with the neurosecretory oxytocin neurones in the paraventricular and supraoptic nuclei. Oxytocin is secreted from the nerve terminal by exocytosis, as a result of increased intracellular Ca^{2+}, due to depolarization of the axon membrane, which opens calcium channels. Oxytocin applied to the oxytocin neurones in the hypothalamus stimulates oxytocin release from the nerve terminals, but the significance of this finding, if any, awaits elucidation.

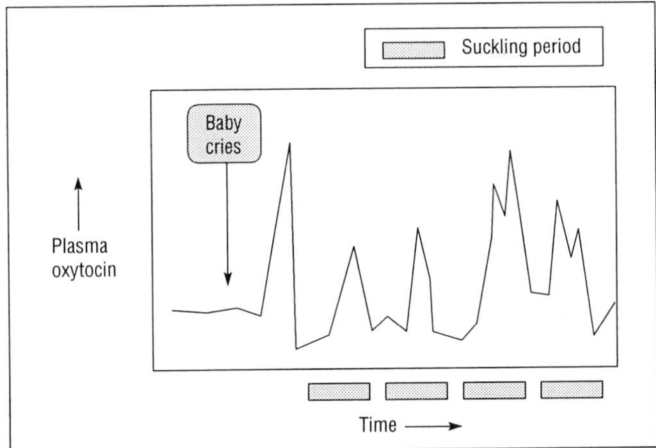

Fig. 31.2 Stimulus to oxytocin release.

ACTIONS

Oxytocin binds to its receptor on target cells, for example, the mammary myoepithelium, or uterine smooth muscle, and activates the phospholipase/inositol triphosphate (PLC/IP_3) system, which increases intracellular calcium and the effect of the hormone is expressed.

Parturition. Oxytocin induces contraction of the smooth muscle of the uterine myometrium, during the last 2–3 weeks of pregnancy. This may be due to a sharp increase in the numbers of oxytocin receptors, whose synthesis is stimulated by the high circulating concentrations of oestrogens present in the third trimester of pregnancy. The trigger for oxytocin receptor synthesis may be the increasing ratio of oestrogen to progesterone, as concentrations of the latter hormone diminish during labour. Oxytocin is released from the posterior pituitary during the course of labour and parturition, possibly as a result of the dilation of the cervix, which sends afferent fibres to the central nervous system. It is not yet known whether the release of oxytocin is the *cause* of the onset of labour in humans.

Milk ejection. Suckling stimulates sensory nerve endings in the nipple and areolus of the breast, and the impulses are conducted along afferent fibres to the spinal cord, where they ascend via the lateral, dorsal and ventral spinothalamic tracts to the midbrain, from where excitatory fibres project directly to the oxytocin neurones in the hypothalamus. Oxytocin binds to receptors on the myoepithelial cells of the mammary tissue, causing contraction of their muscle-like fibres, and this increases intramammary pressure, resulting in ejection of milk from the alveoli into the ducts and out through the teats.

Milk ejection from the breasts can occur even before the suckling reflex is initiated. The sound of a human baby crying may be sufficient to cause milk 'let down'.

Maternal behaviour can be elicited by oxytocin. If virgin rats are administered oxytocin directly into the cerebrospinal fluid, they exhibit maternal behaviour to foster pups. If the rats are ovariectomized, oxytocin no longer has the effect, which can be restored if the ovariectomized rats are first given injections of oestrogen. These experiments suggest that maternal behaviour results from the exposure of the brain to high concentrations of oestrogens, which prime it for the action of oxytocin, which, either as neurotransmitter, or as hormone or both, stimulates maternal behaviour after parturition, and especially during suckling.

Sexual and mating behaviour. Oxytocin is released from the human posterior pituitary during coitus and orgasm, but the significance of this, if any, remains unknown.

32 Vasopressin

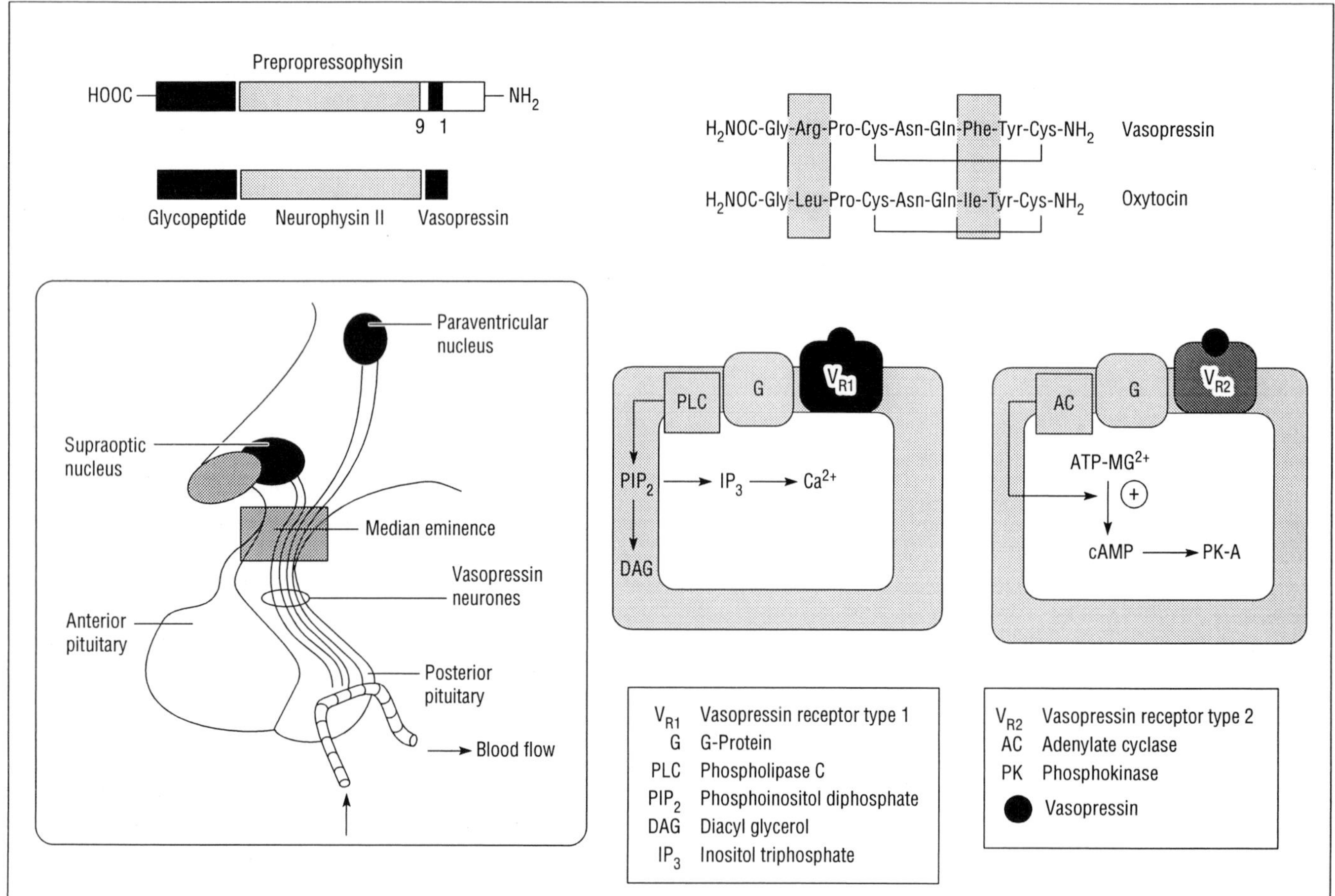

Fig. 32.1 Vasopressin.

BIOSYNTHESIS

Vasopressin, like oxytocin, is a nonapeptide, synthesized mainly in nerve terminals in the magnocellular paraventricular and supraoptic neurones of the hypothalamus. Vasopressin-synthesizing neurones have been identified in other hypothalamic nuclei, such as the suprachiasmatic nucleus, and in extrahypothalamic areas of the limbic system. Axons of vasopressin cell bodies in the hypothalamus project not only to the posterior pituitary, but some are observed to make contact with the fenestrated capillaries of the median eminence portal system, while others project to the spinal cord and other brain centres. Vasopressin may have important roles in brain function (see below), apart from its action on the control of blood volume. In humans, vasopressin is termed arginine vasopressin, as opposed to that in, for example, the pig, where the arginine is replaced by a lysine residue. So far, vasopressin has been discovered only in mammals.

Vasopressin biosynthesis is very similar in principle to that of oxytocin, in that it is packaged in vesicles together with its transport protein, neurophysin II. Prepropressophysin, comprising 166 amino acids, contains the sequence not only of the signal peptide, vasopressin and neurophysin II, but that of a glycopeptide whose role, if any, is unknown. The importance of the neurophysins is highlighted by the discovery that in a mutant strain of rats, the so-called 'Brattleboro' rat, a single nucleotide deletion in the second exon of the gene encoding a very highly conserved region of neurophysin II prevents the translation of vasopressin mRNA. These rats suffer from the equivalent of human diabetes insipidus.

MECHANISM OF ACTION OF VASOPRESSIN

This is through specific receptors on the plasma membrane of the target cell. These have been discovered in many organs, including kidney, pituitary, blood vessels, platelets, liver, the gonads and on tumour cells.

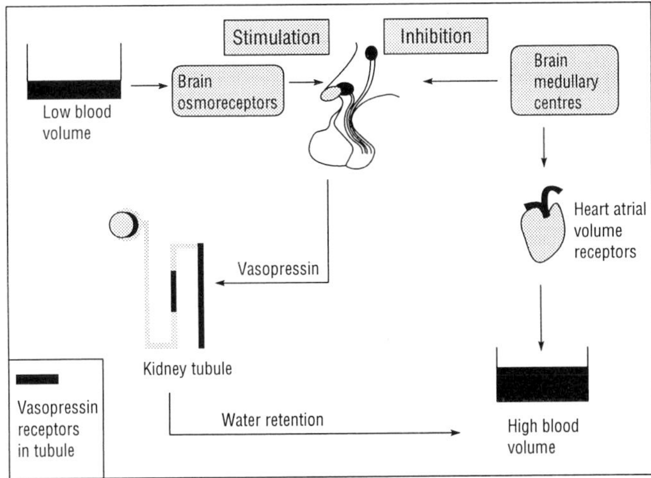

Fig. 32.2 Actions of vasopressin.

VASOPRESSIN RECEPTORS

Two subtypes of vasopressin receptors have been discovered, through the use of synthetic analogues of vasopressin: V_{R1} and V_{R2}. All tissues except the kidney reveal V_{R1}, and are coupled to the IP_3 second messenger system, which mediates the vasopressor action of vasopressin. V_{R2} seem to occur only in the kidney, where they mediate the action of vasopressin on water uptake through cAMP. It now appears that there are many subclasses of V_{R1}.

PHYSIOLOGICAL ACTIONS OF VASOPRESSIN

Kidney. Vasopressin affects the ability of the renal tubules to reabsorb water. The receptors for vasopressin occur principally in the ascending loop of Henle and the collecting ducts, with some in the mesangium (periphery) of the glomerulus. Solutes are powerfully reabsorbed from the loop of Henle, while the walls of the collecting ducts have a variable permeability to water. In the absence of vasopressin, the collecting ducts are impermeable to water, and a hyposmotic urine is voided. In the chronic state, this is diabetes insipidis. When the plasma concenration of vasopressin is high, for example, during dehydration or haemorrhage, the collecting ducts become permeable to water, and a hyperosmotic urine is voided, resulting in a concentration of solutes in plasma. In the healthy individual, vasopressin regulates the development of the osmotic gradient as the tubular filtrate passes through the tubules, and ensures the conservation of water by the body. Vasopressin release from the posterior pituitary is determined principally by blood volume. In the hypothalamus, anatomically near to the paraventricular and supraoptic nuclei, there are osmoreceptors, selectively sensitive to sucrose or sodium ions, which are triggered by a rise in the osmolarity of blood. Vasopressin is released and blood volume rises, which switches off osmoreceptor activity.

Blood pressure. Vasopressin is involved in the regulation of blood pressure, through its effects on blood volume. When this rises, it activates pressure-sensitive receptors in the carotid sinus, the aortic arch and the left atrium, sending afferent messages to the brain stem via the vagus and glossopharangeal nerves, and vasopressin release is inhibited. Vasopressin itself, *within physiological ranges of concentration* in the bloodstream, does not alter blood pressure. (*Vasopressin received its name from the early observation that larger doses than those needed for the antidiuretic effect caused an increase in blood pressure.*)

Adrenocorticotrophic hormone (ACTH) and thyroid-stimulating hormone (TSH) secretion are affected by vasopressin, which reaches the anterior pituitary corticotroph via the portal system. It causes ACTH secretion in its own right as a releasing hormone, and also potentiates the action of corticotrophin-releasing factor (CRF); see page 34. It is not known, however, how important this effect of vasopressin is in the control of ACTH release. Vasopressin, in physiological concentrations, stimulates the release of TSH from the anterior pituitary thyrotroph, and is equipotent with thyrotrophin-releasing hormone (TRH) in this respect. It has also been discovered that vasopressin actually inhibits TRH release, and it has been suggested that centrally released vasopressin may function in the hypothalamus as part of a 'short-loop' negative-feedback regulator of TSH release.

Liver. Vasopressin has a well-known glycogenolytic action in the liver, where the hormone increases the intracellular concentration of Ca^{2+} in hepatocytes. Vasopressin activates the calcium-dependent phosphorylation of the phosphorylase enzyme, which catalyses the conversion of glycogen to glucose phosphate.

Brain. Vasopressin has been shown, after central administration to rats, to inhibit the loss of learned avoidance behaviour, leading to speculation that vasopressin may be involved in memory.

PATHOPHYSIOLOGY

Diabetes insipidis is a permanent condition of water polyuria, due either to a lack of vasopressin production, or to insensitivity of the nephron to vasopressin. The treatment is with stable, long-acting synthetic analogues of vasopressin, such as *desmopressin*. Excessive vasopressin release can occur in the Schwartz–Bartter syndrome, characterized by water retention in the blood with consequent hyponatraemia (low plasma sodium ion concentration). The condition can be caused by vasopressin-secreting tumours, central nervous system disorders such as strokes, drugs such as oxytocin during labour (in high concentrations, oxytocin binds to vasopressin receptors), or by diuretics.

33 Renin–angiotensin–aldosterone system

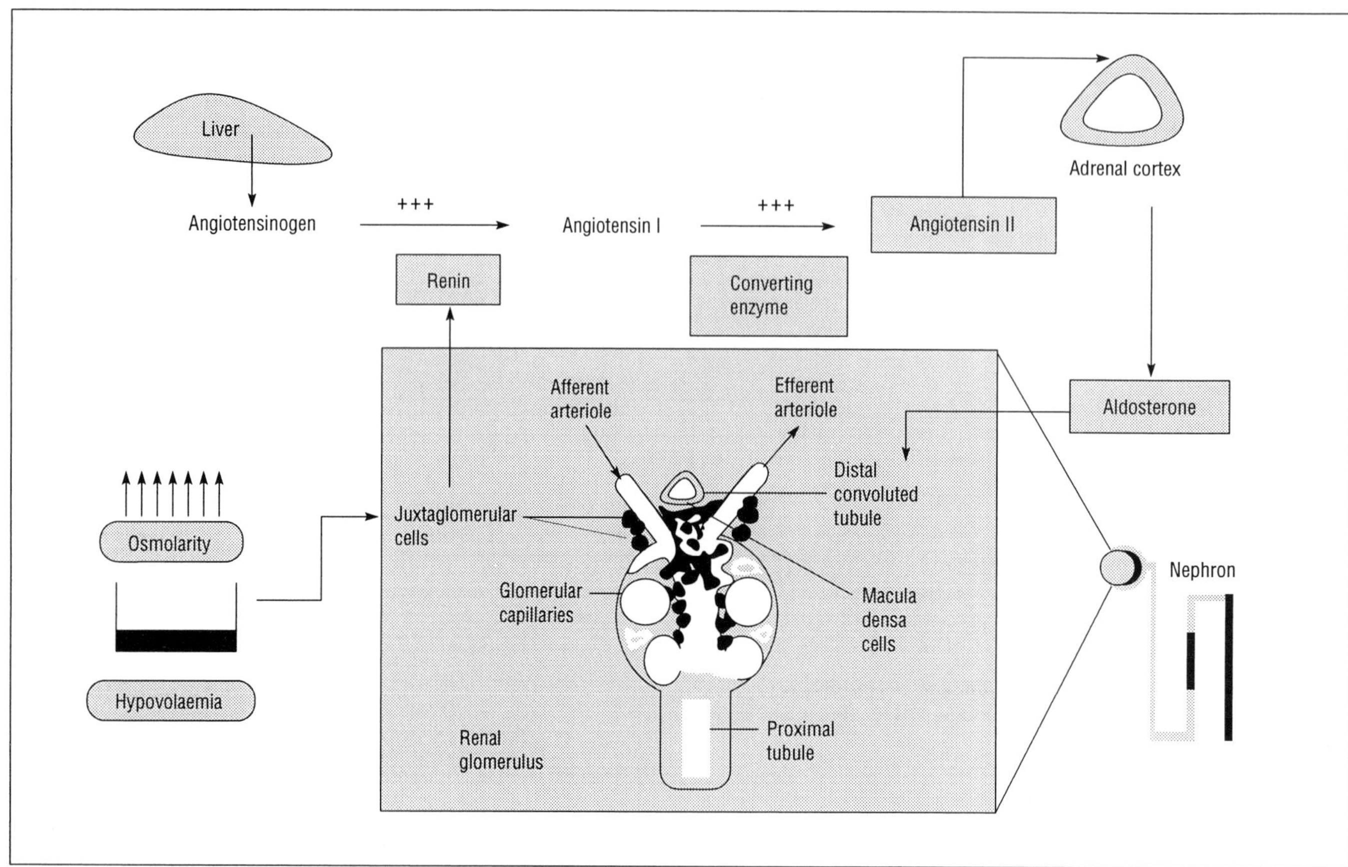

Fig. 33.1 Renin–angiotensin–aldosterone system.

The renin–angiotensin–aldosterone system has a key role in the maintenance of water and electrolyte balance, and in the regulation of arterial blood pressure.

RENIN

Renin is synthesized and stored mainly in the *juxtaglomerular cells* of the kidney. These are located in the walls of the *afferent arterioles* which supply the glomeruli. These arterioles also contain *baroreceptors*, which fire off in response to changes in flow rate and pressure. The cells of the *macula densa* are sensitive to changes in urinary cations such as Ca^{2+}, Na^{2+} and Cl^{-}. The afferent arterioles, the juxtaglomerular cells and the macula densa are together termed the *juxtaglomerular apparatus*.

Release. Renin is an enzyme of molecular weight of about 40 kDa, which is released in response to a rise in blood osmolarity or to hypovolaemia, although there are different theories as to what the physiological stimuli to release are. The theories are:

1 that the macula densa cells monitor changes in cations and pass this information to the adjacent juxtaglomerular cells;
2 that the baroreceptors in the afferent arterioles fire off in response to changes in the mean renal perfusion pressure (the baroreceptors may be part of the juxtaglomerular cells themselves);
3 autonomic innervation of juxtaglomerular cells (sympathetic stimulation releases renin). It is possible that all three theories are significant in the regulation of renin release.

Action. Renin cleaves angiotensinogen to angiotensin I in the plasma and kidney. Angiotensinogen is a globulin of molecular weight of about 60 kDa, which is synthesized continuously in the liver and released in the circulation. Angiotensin I is converted into the biologically active form, the octapeptide *angiotensin II*, by a converting enzyme, which occurs in plasma, vascular endothelial cells, kidney, lung and many other tissues. Angiotensin-converting enzyme (ACE) has another function in the inactivation of a potent vasodilator called bradykinin.

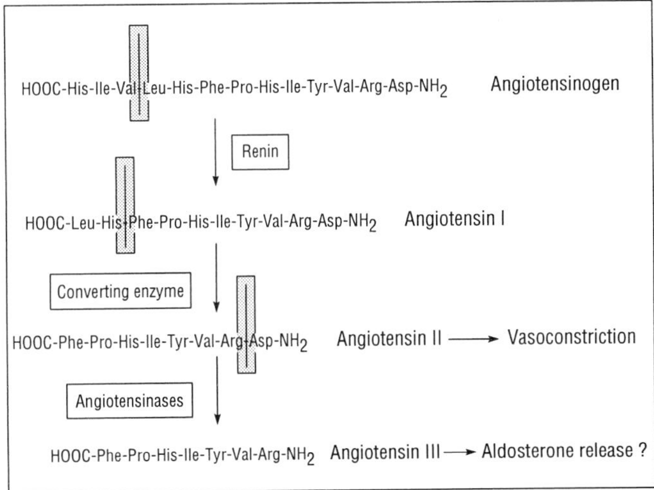

Fig. 33.2 Angiotensin synthesis and actions.

ANGIOTENSIN II

Angiotensin II is the most potent natural vasoconstrictor so far discovered. The hormone is rapidly inactivated by angiotensinase enzymes in the peripheral capillaries. One of the breakdown metabolites, called *angiotensin III*, occurs in large amounts in the adrenal gland, and has been found to stimulate aldosterone release without significant vasopressor effect. Angiotensin III is a heptapeptide, resulting from the removal of the N-terminal aspartic acid from angiotensin II.

Actions of angiotensin II

1 *Vascular smooth muscle and heart.* Angiotensin II has a potent and direct vasoconstrictor effect on vascular muscle, and plays a critical role in the regulation of arterial blood pressure. There are marked regional differences in constrictor responses to angiotensin II in different vascular beds. Blood vessels in the kidney, mesenteric plexus and the skin are highly responsive to angiotensin II, while those in the brain, lungs and skeletal muscle respond less to administered peptide. In the heart, angiotensin II acts on atrial and ventricular myocytes during the plateau phase of the action potential, to increase Ca^{2+} entry through voltage-gated channels, thereby prolonging the action potential, which increases the force of contraction of the heart.
2 *Kidney.* Angiotensin II regulates glomerular permeability, tubular Na^+ and water reabsorption and renal haemodynamics. Angiotensin II has three important renal actions.

(a) It constricts the renal arterioles, especially the efferent arterioles, which lowers the glomerular filtration rate proportionately more than renal blood flow. This causes an increase in the osmolarity of blood feeding into the peritubular capillaries, which drives solutes and water back into the tubular cell and thence to the bloodstream.

(b) Angiotensin II has been shown to constrict glomerular mesangial cells, which also contributes to the fall in glomerular filtration rate.

(c) Angiotensin II has a direct action on the tubule cells to stimulate Na^+ reabsorption.

3 *Adrenal cortex.* Angiotensin II alone, or through conversion to angiotensin III, acts on the glomerulosa cells to increase aldosterone synthesis.
4 *Nervous system.* Angiotensin II binds to specific presynaptic receptors on sympathetic nerve terminals to enhance noradrenaline release. It has been shown to depolarize adrenal medullary chromaffin cells, causing release of adrenaline, and when injected directly into the brain, causes an increase in salt and thirst appetite. Angiotensin stimulates vasopressin release from the posterior pituitary gland, an effect potentiated by dehydration.
5 Angiotensin II stimulates Na^+ and water absorption from the lumen of the gastrointestinal tract (GIT) at low doses. During dehydration, haemorrhage, or salt loss, angiotensin II acts on the small intestine to limit loss, while aldosterone acts predominantly upon the large intestine to limit loss.
6 *Cell proliferation.* Angiotensin II has been shown to have trophic effects on smooth muscle vascular cells, fibroblasts, adrenocortical cells and human fetal kidney mesangial cells. The peptide appears to stimulate the production of specific proteins such as alpha-actin, and may play a role in repair following vascular injury.

Angiotensin II receptor subtypes have been discovered using different analogues of angiotensin II. The angiotensin I receptor, acting through G proteins and the IP_3 second messenger system, mediates the increase in blood pressure in extracellular volume and cell proliferation. The angiotensin II receptor may mediate cell proliferation.

Tissue distribution of receptor subtypes. Aortic smooth muscle cells, GIT, kidney, liver, lung, placenta and urinary bladder express exclusively angiotensin I receptors. Both angiotensin I and angiotensin II receptors are expressed in the brain, where angiotensin I receptors may mediate the central actions of angiotensin II on blood pressure, water and electrolyte balance, the renal arterioles, adrenal cells, heart and uterus. There is evidence for the existence of even more subtypes of angiotensin II receptors.

34 The pineal gland

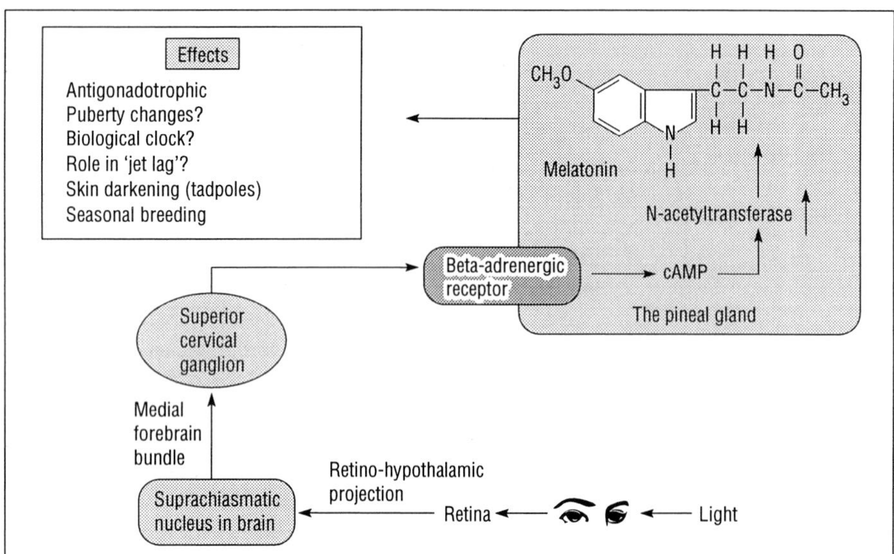

Fig. 34.1 Melatonin release and actions.

The pineal gland is an endocrine organ, secreting the hormone *melatonin*, and possibly others. In humans, the pineal is a pine-shaped body (hence its name), weighing about 175 mg, which invaginates from the roof of the diencephalon, moving away from the third ventricle, and is attached to the brain by a stalk. The gland is composed of pinealocyte cells, which contain darkly staining material and glycogen, fibroblasts and glial cells. It is innervated by postganglionic fibres which originate in the superior cervical ganglion. During the second decade of life, the gland starts to calcify; nevertheless, there is no evidence that calcification is associated with a loss of pineal activity through life.

Although known from antiquity, the function of the pineal in humans has never been fully ascertained. The first indication that the pineal had a function was the discovery that a tumour which destroyed the pineal was associated with precocious puberty in a boy. Subsequently, the hormone melatonin (*N*-acetyl-5-methoxytryptamine) was isolated from the pineal.

MELATONIN

Melatonin is synthesized from dietary tryptophan, which is first converted to 5-hydroxytryptamine (5HT), and then to melatonin. Biosynthesis of melatonin in the rat pineal increases dramatically at night, when the activity of the enzyme *N*-acetyltransferase is increased up to one hundredfold. Enzyme activity in the pineal is rapidly depressed by light. Since 5HT is the substrate for melatonin synthesis, pineal concentrations of 5HT fall during periods of darkness. The neural pathway from the eyes to the pineal is via the suprachiasmatic nucleus, from which impulses are relayed through the medial forebrain bundle to the upper thoracic spinal cord and out to the superior cervical ganglia. Postganglionic sympathetic fibres project directly to the pineal gland. These release noradrenaline, which acts on pinealocyte beta-receptors. The suprachiasmatic nucleus has been proposed as a form of biological clock, mediating brain rhythms (see below), and would thus be a candidate regulator of pineal activity.

The secretion of melatonin has been demonstrated, since pinealectomy reduces plasma concentrations of the hormone. Plasma concentrations of melatonin are highest at the dark midpoint, and lowest at midday.

The actions of melatonin are still obscure, but there is evidence that the hormone acts both in the brain and the peripheral organs. In the brain, administered melatonin induces sleep with slow electroencephalograph (EEG) activity and prolongs the duration of barbiturate-induced sleep. It has been suggested that administration of melatonin is helpful in lessening the symptoms of jet-lag.

Melatonin exerts an *antigonadotrophic action*, which means that it causes gonadal regression. This has been found after implanting melatonin directly into the mouse hypothalamus, presumably inhibiting gonadotrophin-releasing hormone (GnRH) release. There is no evidence from human studies that melatonin affects the GnRH-induced release of luteinizing hormone (LH) and follicle-stimulating hormone (FSH). Melatonin has been shown to inhibit testicular testosterone biosynthesis, and pinealectomy of castrated rats enhances the growth response of the ventral prostate gland to testosterone. Melatonin may be involved in puberty, since plasma concentrations of the hormone decrease in males and females until the end of puberty (see below).

Melatonin and the pineal have a role in *seasonal breeding* in animals. In the hamster, for example, which breeds seasonally in the wild and hibernates, there is a daily rhythm of pineal melatonin synthesis, which is eliminated after removal of the superior cervical ganglion. In long, dark periods, melatonin synthesis is increased, and this is associated with gonadal atrophy. There is evidence that during short days, when melatonin production increases, the hypothalamic–pituitary system becomes very much more sensitive to the negative-feedback effects of gonadal steroid hormones on gonadotrophin production. This phenomenon may be relevant to theories of puberty onset in humans, since it has been postulated that puberty may be due to a change in the sensitivity of the hypothalamus to the negative-feedback effect of steroid hormones (see page 45).

The importance of melatonin in seasonal breeding has been demonstrated in ewes, when the administration of supplemental daily doses of melatonin in the late afternoon during mid-summer, advanced the onset of reproductive activity. In other words, the additional melatonin tricked the brain into thinking that the day length had shortened.

Biological rhythms are known to exist, but their regulation and significance are largely a mystery. The rhythms of glucocorticoid production have already been dealt with (page 37), and it seems that some physiological, and especially endocrine rhythms are linked to environmental changes or time cues (sometimes referred to in the literature as 'zeitgebers'). One of the most obvious cues is that of light. The circadian rhythms of 24 hours are generated in the brain by a biological clock that transmits signals periodically to other brain areas, including the pineal. Cycles of light and possibly temperature entrain the signal generator to synchronize with the external environment. In the brain, the suprachiasmatic nucleus (SCN) is generally accepted to be the biological clock, generating its rhythmic discharges autonomously, but tuned to the external environment.

Evidence for the SCN being the biological clock comes from experiments in which the SCN was removed from an animal's brain and cultured *in vitro*, and the explant continued to generate regular, periodic electrical discharges. *In vivo*, the SCN shows a rhythmicity of glucose utilization. Biological rhythms, in general, are the regular occurrence of chemical or electrical events. Removal of the SCN from an animal's brain abolishes rhythms of brain electrical discharges and deletes rhythms of behaviour. These rhythms are restored if fragments of fetal SCN-containing tissue are implanted into the animal's brain. It has also been found that the pregnant mother trains the biological clocks of her fetuses to synchronize with her own, suggesting an endocrine maternal message whose release is dictated by the maternal SCN. This maternal training of fetal rhythms persists even in the absence of a maternal pineal gland.

35 Insulin: I

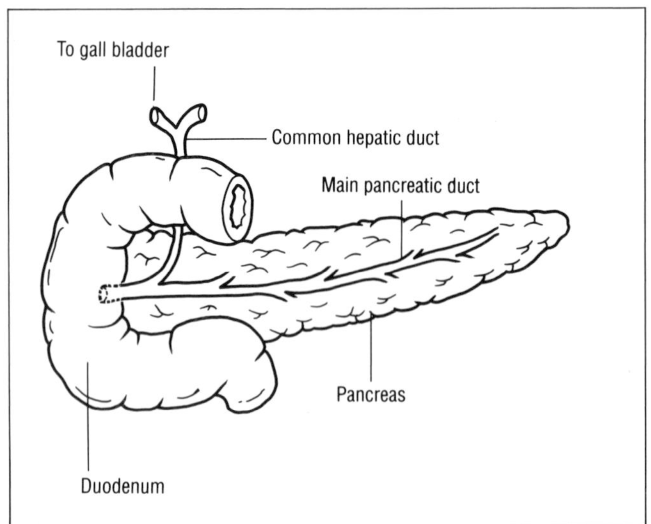

Fig. 35.1 The pancreas.

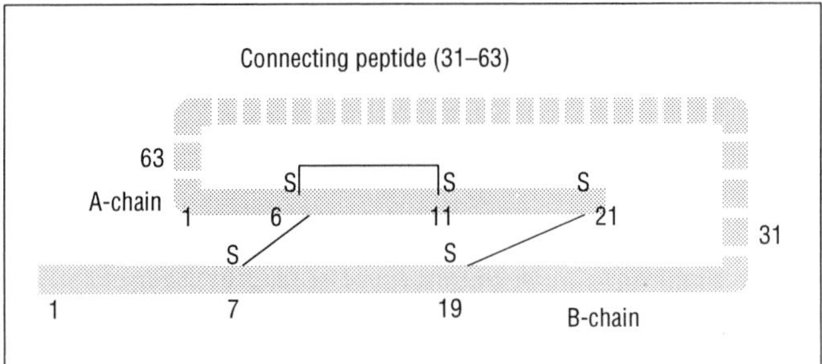

Fig. 35.2 Structure of porcine insulin.

The pancreas is a gland consisting of two major tissue types, namely the *acini*, which secrete digestive juices into the duodenum, and the *islets of Langerhans*, which secrete insulin and glucagon directly into the bloodstream, and are therefore truly endocrine. The human pancreas has between 1–2 million islets, each organized around small capillaries into which the hormones are secreted. The islets can be distinguished by differential staining techniques into three types: A, B and D (sometimes called alpha, beta and delta). The B cells, which constitute about 60% of the islet cells, lie towards the middle of the islet and secrete *insulin*. The A cells secrete *glucagon* and the D cells secrete *somatostatin*. Another cell type, called the PP cell, secretes a substance called pancreatic polypeptide. A physiological role for pancreatic polypeptide has not yet been identified with certainty.

INSULIN

Insulin is the hormone secreted by the B cells of the islets of Langerhans in the pancreas. It is a protein, it was the first to be crystallized and it was the first protein whose primary structure was determined. Insulin is still the only treatment for juvenile onset diabetes mellitus, a disease which results from the destruction of pancreatic B cells.

Chemistry. Insulin consists of two chains, an A-chain of 21 amino acids, and a B-chain of 30 amino acids, linked by two disulphide bridges (A7–B7 and A20–B19). Another disulphide bridge links 6–11 on the A-chain. Human and porcine (pig) insulin differ only in respect of one residue (B30), and beef insulin differs from human insulin at A8 and A10. The primary structure of the insulin molecule has been relatively well preserved throughout evolution. Insulin can exist as a monomer (molecular weight of 6 kDa), the form in which it predominantly circulates. It can dimerize to form a dimer of molecular weight of 12 kDa, and three dimers can aggregate in the presence of two zinc atoms to form a hexamer of molecular weight 36 kDa.

Biosynthesis. Insulin is cleaved from a precursor called proinsulin (molecular weight of 9 kDa). Proinsulin, in turn, is derived from an even larger precursor, preproinsulin, which is synthesized in the rough endoplasmic reticulum. Proinsulin is a continuous chain which starts at the N-terminal end of the B-chain and terminates at the C-terminal end of the A-chain. A connecting peptide is interposed between the C-terminal end of the B-chain and the N-terminal end of the A-chain. In the Golgi apparatus and the storage granules, a converting enzyme cleaves proinsulin to yield insulin. The adult human pancreas contains about 5 mg of stored insulin. In humans, the gene coding for insulin is located on the short arm of chromosome 11.

Secretion of insulin. Insulin synthesis and secretion is stimulated by glucose, which stimulates the B cell to take up extracellular calcium (Ca^{2+}). The cation appears to trigger a contractile mechanism, whereby the microtubules participate in the movement of insulin-containing granules towards the cell membrane, where granules fuse and the granule contents are released into the extracellular space by exocytosis. Insulin secretion in response to a sudden rise in circulating glucose occurs in a biphasic fashion: there is an immediate release of stored insulin, lasting less than a minute, followed by a more sustained release of both stored and newly synthesized insulin. A great many other substances stimulate insulin release, but not all elicit a biphasic release pattern. Carbohydrates, most amino acids and, to a lesser extent, fatty acids and ketones, all stimulate insulin release. Although a number of gut hormones can stimulate insulin release, the physiological significance of this, if any, is unknown. Glucagon, which is synthesized in the pancreatic A cells, stimulates insulin release by direct action on the B cells.

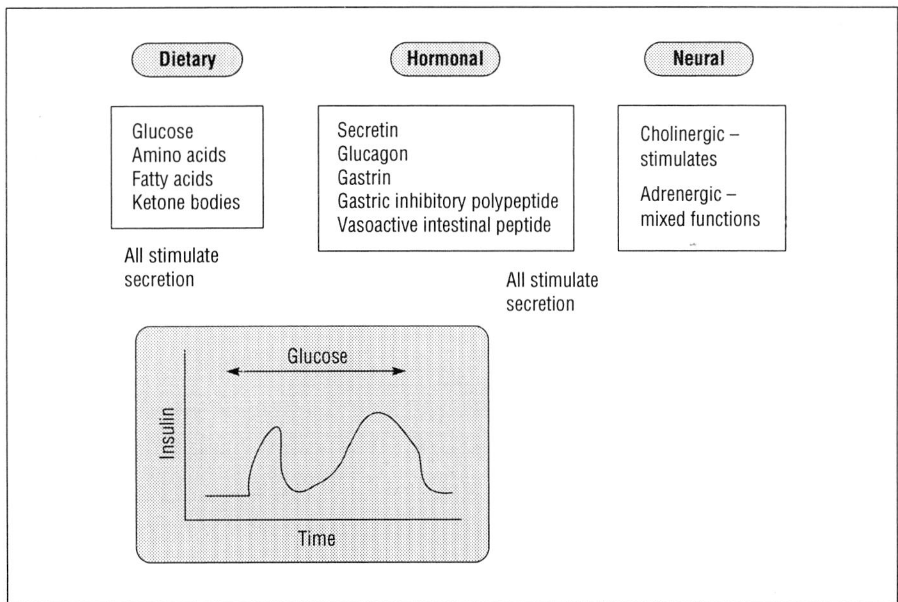

Fig. 35.3 Control of insulin secretion.

Insulin release is also affected by the nervous system and by neurotransmitters. Acetylcholine stimulates insulin release, as does adrenaline, acting on beta receptors. Stimulation of alpha-receptors, on the other hand, causes an inhibition of insulin release. Stimulation of different areas of the hypothalamus in experimental animals has different effects on insulin release. For example, electrical stimulation of the ventrolateral region stimulates insulin release, while electrical stimulation of the ventromedial region inhibits insulin release. Note that the basal secretion of insulin is also affected by neurotransmitters. It has been found that drugs which block adrenergic alpha receptors increase basal insulin tone, while drugs which block beta receptors reduce basal insulin tone.

Insulin metabolism. Insulin circulates as a monomer, unbound to plasma proteins. It is filtered by the glomeruli, but is almost completely reabsorbed in the proximal tubules, and is degraded by the kidneys.

The liver removes about half the hepatic portal insulin that passes through it. The half-life of insulin in plasma is about 5 minutes. Proinsulin, which is also released with insulin, has a longer half-life (about 20 minutes). Proinsulin is not cleaved to insulin in the plasma. Although the liver and kidneys are the major sites of insulin degradation, virtually all the tissues of the body can break down the hormone. Insulin can be degraded extracellularly, and also intracellularly, after it has bound to its receptor and become internalized in the cell.

36 Insulin: II

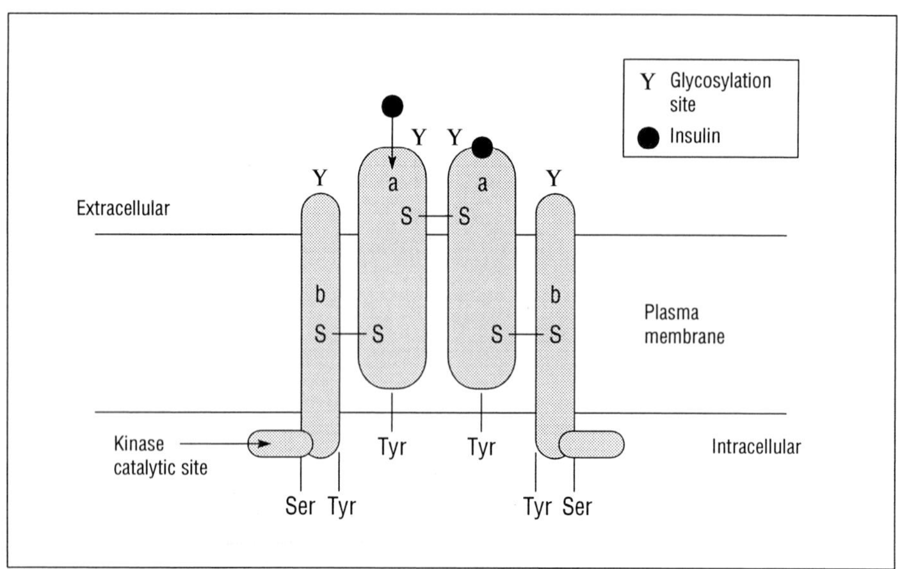

Fig. 36.1 Insulin-receptor structure.

MECHANISM OF ACTION OF INSULIN

The actions of insulin are mediated by a specific receptor located on the plasma membrane of the cell.

The insulin receptor consists of subunits; it has two alpha subunits and two beta subunits, which are linked covalently to each other by disulphide bridges. The alpha subunits are extracellular, and contain the insulin-binding sites. The beta subunits span the membrane, and transduce the binding of insulin to the alpha subunits into an intracellular signal. When insulin binds to the receptor site, this interaction is somehow transmitted to the intracellular domain of the beta subunit. This subunit becomes autophosphorylated, which in turn activates its own protein kinases, resulting in an intracellular cascade of phosphorylation and dephosphorylation reactions through which the actions of insulin are expressed.

Despite an intensive search, no second messenger for insulin has been identified.

A link between the insulin receptor and the rest of the phosphorylation cascade may be a protein called insulin receptor substrate (IRS-1). IRS-1 is an intracellular protein which is tyrosine phosphorylated, and this confers on IRS-1 the ability to bind another set of signalling proteins that contain signalling domains, the SH2 domains. It is thought that IRS-1 is a sort of 'docking' protein for the SH2-containing signalling proteins. An important action of insulin is the conversion of glucose into glycogen, and this reaction is controlled by the enzyme glycogen synthetase, which is inactive in the phosphorylated state, and activated by dephosphorylation. Hepatic phosphorylase, on the other hand, is activated by phosphorylation. Hepatic phosphorylase activates glycogenolysis. It has been suggested that insulin exerts its action on glycogen metabolism through its inhibition of phosphorylation of both these enzymes, possibly through the mechanism involving SH2 domains.

Receptor action and glucose transporters. When the receptor binds insulin, the receptor is autophosphorylated through Mg^{2+}/ATP-dependent reactions, and the complex stimulates the cellular uptake of glucose, a major physiological action of insulin. Glucose is taken into the cell by glucose transporters, through a process of facilitated diffusion. The transporters can transfer glucose and other sugars across the cell membrane down a chemical concentration gradient. Glucose transporters vary in structure and ionic requirements from tissue to tissue.

After the receptor binds insulin, the hormone–receptor complex leaves the membrane through a process of endocytosis and enters the cell. After binding to the receptor, the complex becomes encapsulated in a coated pit, formed by invagination and fusion of the cell surface. Once inside the cell, the pit becomes progressively uncoated to form what is called an endosome. The endosome releases the receptor and insulin, the former being mainly recycled to the membrane, and insulin being degraded. The process of *receptor internalization* may provide a means of regulating the effects of insulin by limiting the numbers of receptors available for binding to the hormone. This effectively downregulates the insulin receptor.

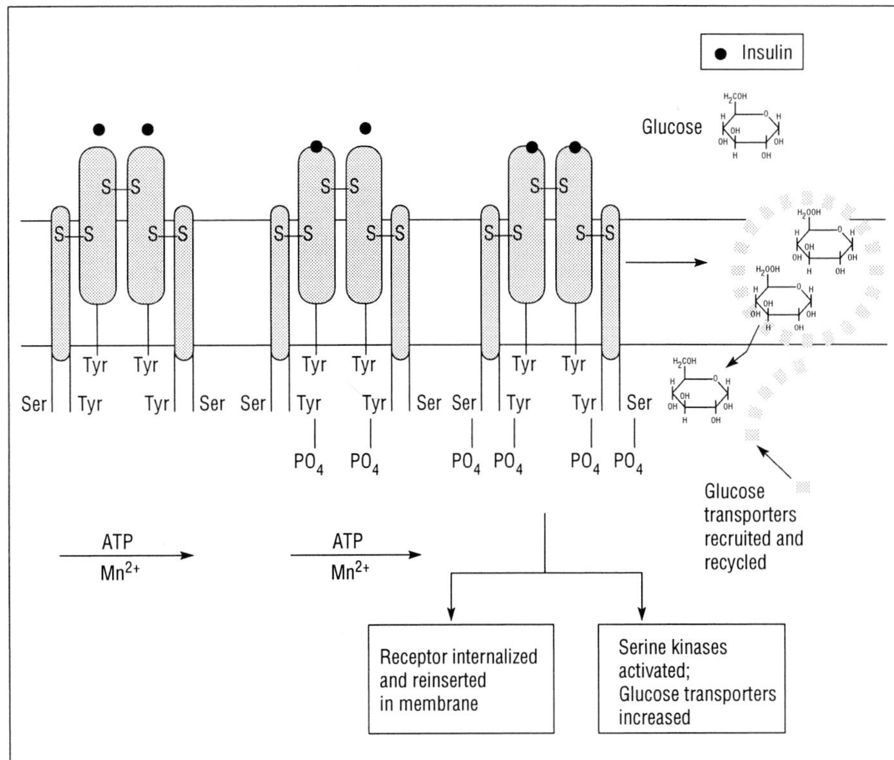

Fig. 36.2 Insulin-receptor dynamics.

37 Insulin: III

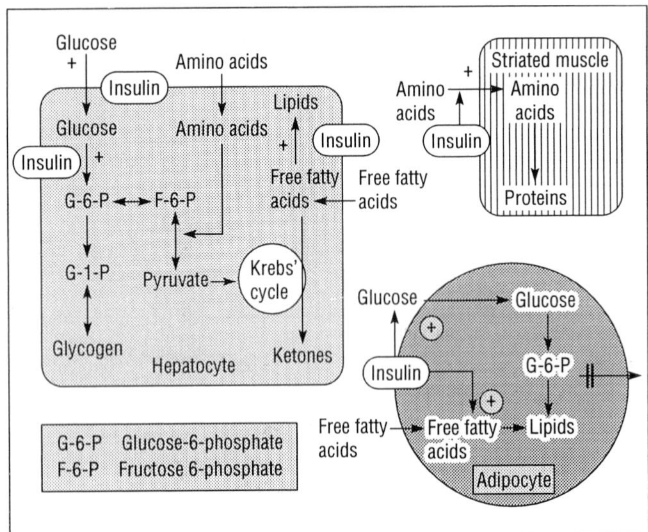

Fig. 37.1 Insulin action.

INSULIN EFFECTS

When glucose enters the circulation, through a meal for example, insulin is released immediately from the pancreatic islets. Insulin removes glucose from the circulation and promotes its conversion to glycogen and lipids. Insulin promotes the conversion of fatty acids to lipids, and the uptake of amino acids into liver and skeletal muscle, where they are elaborated into protein. Insulin is thus an anabolic hormone.

Liver. The liver is the major organ in which gluconeogenesis and ketogenesis occur. Lipid and protein production also take place in the liver. When insulin binds to the liver insulin receptor, it stimulates a number of enzymes involved in glycogen production, including glycogen synthetase, which catalyses the formation of glycogen. Glycogen within the hepatocyte is a major source of stored carbohydrate. Glycogen is also stored in smaller amounts in skeletal muscle and other cells which need to mobilize energy stores rapidly. Within the cell, glucose is also converted into glucose-6-phosphate (G6P), which is unable to leave the cell, since the plasma membrane is impermeable to phosphoric acid esters. This creates a concentration gradient, and more glucose moves into the cell.

Fat. Approximately 90% of stored glucose is in the form of lipids. The adipocyte is therefore an important site of insulin action. Insulin is required for the activation of the enzyme lipoprotein lipase. If insulin is absent, lipoproteins accumulate in the circulation. Insulin also opposes the action of glucagon (see page 83), which promotes the production of the *ketone bodies*. The ketone bodies, acetone, acetoacetic acid and beta-hydroxybutyric acid, are an energy source for muscle and brain, especially during prolonged fasting. They are derived from lipids, and are produced in conditions of insulin lack (see below). The ketone bodies inhibit the oxidation of glucose and of fatty acids, which results in the preferential use of the ketone bodies as a source of energy. When their rate of production exceeds their rate of utilization, a condition known as keto-acidosis will result.

Muscle. Insulin stimulates the uptake of amino acids into skeletal muscle, and increases the incorporation of amino acids into proteins. These two actions are independent of insulin's action on glucose transport into the cell.

Other actions of insulin include its role as a growth factor in the mammary gland, which becomes highly sensitive to insulin during pregnancy and lactation. Although the brain does not appear to require insulin, there are receptors for insulin in specific brain areas, including parts of the hypothalamus which contain the satiety centre. Insulin stimulates the membrane ATPase in lymphocytes, and the uptake of amino acids by thymocytes, although the physiological significance of this remains unknown.

Insulin lack creates a profoundly catabolic state, sometimes termed an insulinopenic syndrome. Without insulin, glucose is not taken up by the tissues, and hyperglycaemia results. The cells are deprived of an energy source and respond by glycogenolysis, gluconeogenesis and lipolysis to generate glucose for energy. This exacerbates the hyperglycaemia, and creates an acidosis through the increased production of ketone bodies, which can prove fatal. The breakdown of body proteins and fats results in weight loss, also called wasting, and the acidosis produces vasodilatation and hypothermia. The patient hyperventilates to blow off the acidosis in the form of carbon dioxide. The decreased anabolic state and hyperglycaemia cause fatigue.

Glucose is excreted in the urine, in the form of diuresis, which in turn results in loss of body fluids and salts. The patient becomes dehydrated, is constantly thirsty and drinks copious volumes of water (polydipsia). The patient will eventually fall into a coma, the aetiology of which is not fully understood, but which may result from the combined effects of hyperketonaemia, including dehydration, hyperosmolarity due to hyperglycaemia and problems within the cerebral microcirculation.

Pancreatic pathophysiology. Abnormal insulin production, or an abnormal cellular response to insulin may produce the symptoms outlined above.

Insulin-dependent diabetes mellitis (IDDM) (sometimes called Type I) most often presents itself in juveniles and adults below the age of 40, and is more prevalent in the white population. There may be a genetic disposition to IDDM, and the disease may be an autoimmune one, since autoantibodies to pancreatic

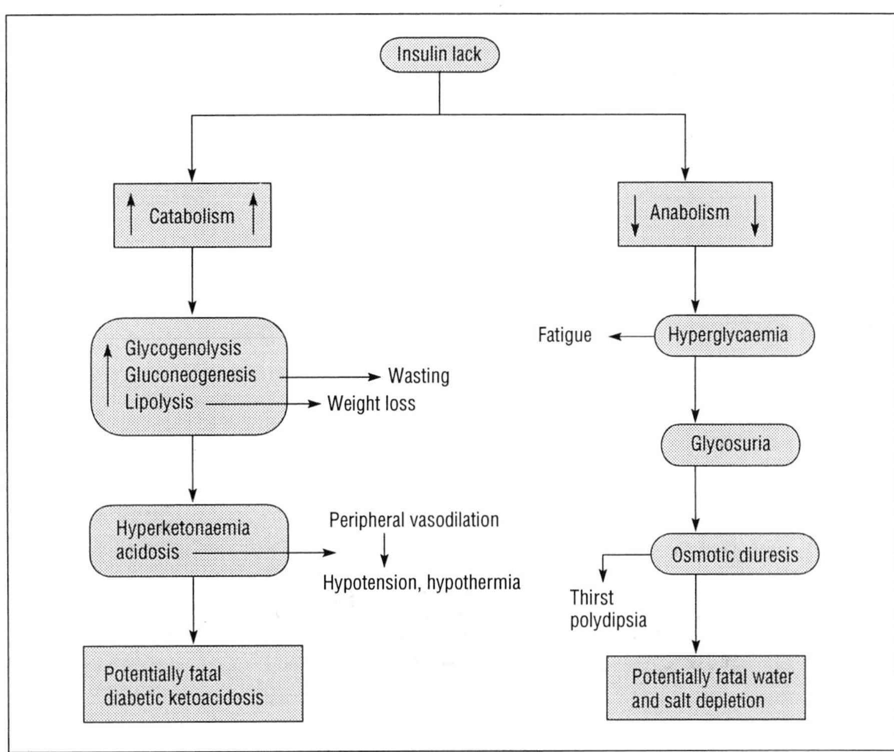

Fig. 37.2 Insulin lack.

islet cells have been detected in the circulation of patients, and the disease is associated with particular human leucocyte antigen (HLA) profiles. Another theory holds that the disease is caused by a virus infection resulting in B-cell alteration. IDDM is caused by the destruction of the B cells, and the patient is completely dependent on insulin for survival.

Non-insulin dependent diabetes mellitis (NIDDM) is also referred to as Type 2 diabetes, and was commonly called adult-onset diabetes. This is the most common form of diabetes, occurring in approximately 85% of patients. Patients present with symptoms of insulin deficiency, sometimes together with a reduced cellular responsiveness to the hormone. The disease occurs more commonly in middle-aged patients, and appears to be genetically linked, although it is not associated with any particular HLA profiles. Obesity and a certain form of lifestyle, linked to poor or inappropriate nutrition, are known risk factors for the development of NIDDM. Patients are given dietary advice, and, if necessary, treated with insulin and/or oral sulphonylurea drugs such as *glibenclamide*, which cause insulin release from the pancreas. Clearly, these drugs are useless in IDDM, since they require a functioning pancreatic B cell.

Gestational diabetes. Some patients present with diabetes during pregnancy, in the form of an abnormal response to the glucose tolerance test, which is a test in which the patient is given a non-physiological intravenous injection of glucose, and the rate of decline of plasma glucose is measured.

Hyperinsulinaemia may result from excessive administration of insulin, resulting in hypoglycaemia, which produces clear signs of brain glucose starvation, including confusion, convulsions and coma. Pancreatic insulin-secreting tumours will also produce these symptoms.

38 Glucagon

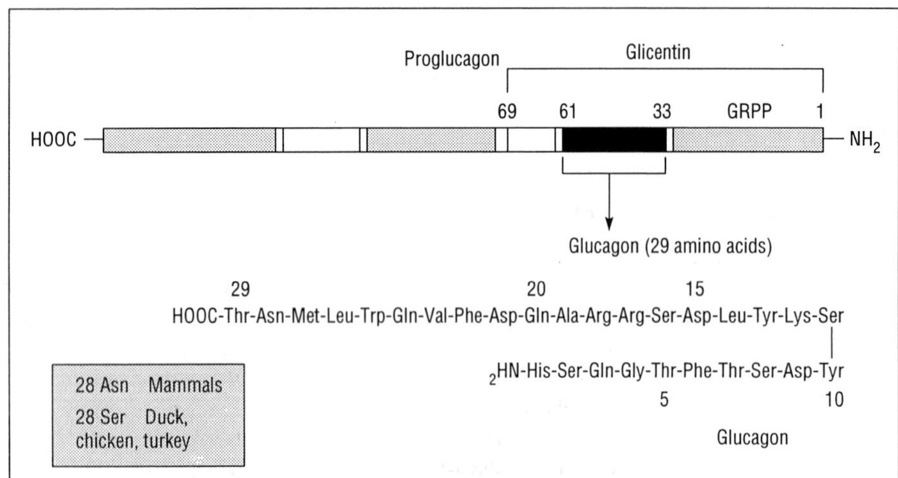

Fig. 38.1 Glucagon synthesis.

BIOSYNTHESIS, STORAGE AND SECRETION

Glucagon is synthesized principally in the pancreatic A cell, and is cleaved from a much larger precurser molecule, preproglucagon (179 amino acids in humans). The preproglucagon gene in humans is located on chromosome 2. Preproglucagon yields proglucagon. The N-terminal fragment of proglucagon is termed glicentin-related polypeptide fragment (GRPP), so-called because it contains glicentin (glucagon-like immunoreactivity-1), an intestinal glucagon sequence-containing polypeptide. GRPP and glucagon are stored together in the cell in granules, and released together in approximately equimolar quantities. Both these peptide sequences are also stored and released from cells in the gut, and glucagon and GRPP form part of a larger family of gut hormones (see page 85). The glucagon content of a healthy human adult pancreas ranges from about 3–5 μg/g of net pancreas weight.

Chemically, glucagon is a polypeptide of molecular weight of about 3.5 kDa, consisting of 29 amino acids. The amino acid sequence of glucagon has been well conserved throughout evolution, and the whole amino ácid is required for full biological activity. If the N-terminal histidine is replaced, the molecule loses biological activity. Insulin, on the other hand, depends for its action more on the integrity of its three-dimensional structure,

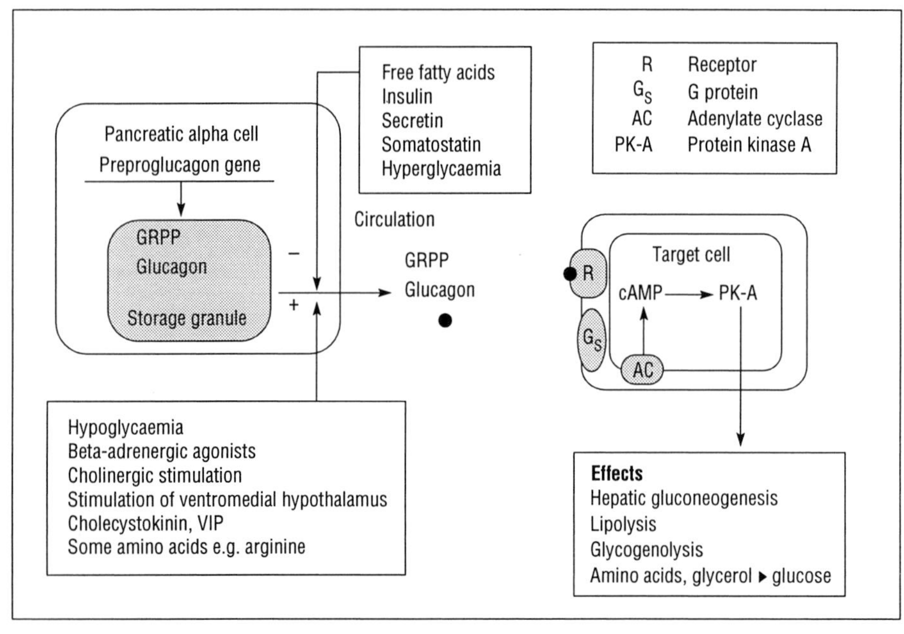

Fig. 38.2 Glucagon.

rather than on an absolute dependence on amino acid sequence. Unlike insulin, glucagon does not have a stable three-dimensional structure in physiological solutions, but may acquire this when it binds to its receptor.

Glucagon is rapidly secreted when plasma glucose concentrations fall, and secretion is inhibited when glucose concentrations rise. Secretion is inhibited also by other energy substrates, such as ketone bodies and fatty acids. Amino acids, particularly arginine, stimulate glucagon secretion (as they do insulin). In this situation, where both insulin and glucagon are released simultaneously, the effect may be to allow insulin to promote protein synthesis without a disturbance of normal glucose homeostasis.

Insulin inhibits glucagon secretion, perhaps through a paracrine reciprocal interaction between the pancreatic A and B cells. Glucagon secretion is affected by gut hormones (see page 85), being stimulated by cholecystokinin (CCK) and vasointestinal peptide (VIP). Somatostatin, another hormone secreted by, among many other tissues, the pancreas, inhibits the secretion of both glucagon and insulin.

The nervous system mediates glucagon release, which is effected by cholinergic and beta-adrenergic stimulation. Electrical stimulation of the ventromedial hypothalamus in experimental animals increases glucagon release.

Once released into the circulation, glucagon circulates unbound to any plasma protein, and exists in several forms, which creates problems when measuring glucagon by radioimmunoassay (RIA), since many forms cross-react with the antibodies used in RIA. The hormone has a short half-life of about 5 minutes, being rapidly degraded, especially in the kidney and liver. In the liver, glucagon binds to a specific membrane receptor, after which it is degraded, a degradation process apparently peculiar to glucagon.

MECHANISM OF ACTION

Glucagon binds to a membrane receptor on the target cell, and activates the adenylate cyclase second messenger system. It was through the study of glucagon action on gluconeogenesis that the second messenger system of cellular response was first discovered.

EFFECTS OF GLUCAGON

Glucagon has the opposite effects to those exerted by insulin. In the *liver*, the hormone promotes the formation of glucose the breakdown of glycogen. Glucagon, through cAMP, blocks the enzyme cascade leading to glycogen at the level of the enzyme activities between fructose-6-phosphate and fructose-1,6-diphosphate, and between pyruvate and phosphoenolpyruvate. The glycolytic action of glucagon is essential for maintaining short-term glucose blood levels, especially in the fed state, when glycogen stores are high. In the liver, glucagon promotes the conversion of amino acids to glucose. The hormone also promotes the conversion of free fatty acids to ketone bodies.

Within the *hepatocyte*, glucagon is lipolytic, liberating free fatty acids and glycerol, but its actions on the hepatocyte may only be significant when insulin concentrations are low, since insulin is a very potent inhibitor of hepatocyte lipolysis.

39 Gastrointestinal hormones

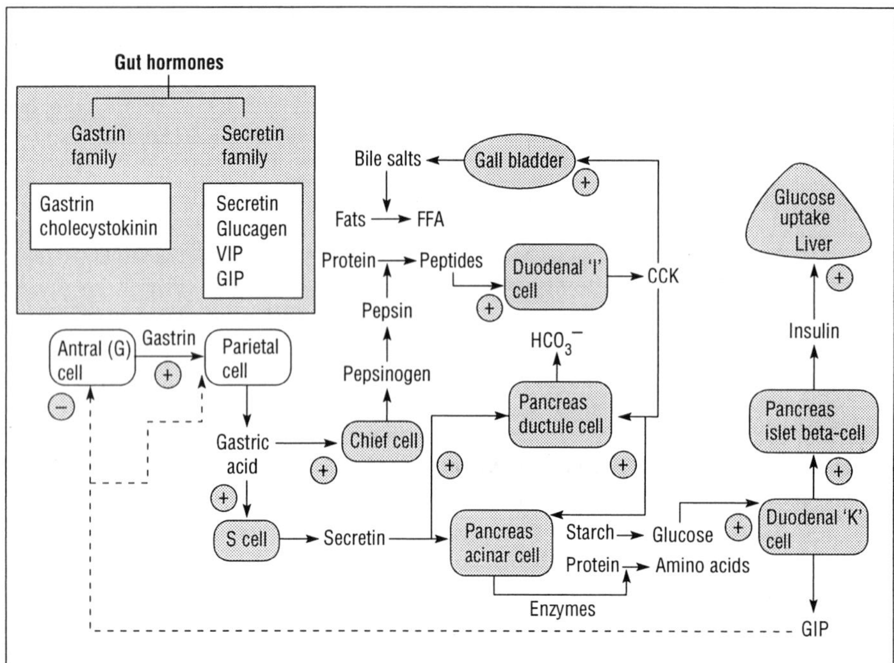

Fig. 39.1 Gut hormones.

Gastrointestinal hormones form a large and not yet completely characterized group of substances, widely scattered throughout the gastrointestinal tract (GIT). Their main functions are to ensure the digestion of food and its movement along the GIT. They are principally peptides, four of which are known to be endocrine hormones: cholecystokinin (CCK), gastrin, gastric inhibitory peptide (GIP) and secretin, which was the first hormone to be discovered in 1902 by Bayliss and Starling. Very many peptides are synthesized by GIT cells, but their role as hormones awaits confirmation. The GIT hormones release enzymes necessary for digestion; they enhance enzyme activity by stimulating the release of bile acids, which provide an optimal acid pH for many enzymes, and the bile salts, which enable the emulsification of dietary fats, thus facilitating their passage into the bloodstream; some alter GIT motility. Two important pancreatic hormones, namely insulin and glucagon, have already been covered. The pancreas, through its exocrine acinar cells (exocrine glands have ducts), secretes enzymes and ions, notably bicarbonate, which play an important part in digestion.

BIOSYNTHESIS, CHEMISTRY AND RELEASE OF GASTROINTESTINAL TRACT HORMONES

The GIT hormones are synthesized in 'clear' cells, named because of their selective staining with silver salts, and are widely diffused throughout the gut, thus giving rise to the *DES*, or diffuse endocrine system of the gut. As in the pancreas, gut cells have been arbitrarily named, for example, G cells (gastrin-secreting), S cells (secretin-secreting), D cells (somatostatin-secreting), K cells (GIP-secreting), and I cells (CCK-secreting). The GIT hormones are conveniently grouped according to their structural similarities into two main *families*.

The *secretin family* of peptides, namely secretin, glucagon, VIP and GIP share sequence homology in many amino acids. Secretin and glucagon have 14 amino acids in common. The *gastrin family* is so-called because gastrin and CCK have identical C-terminal sequences of the first five amino acids.

Gastrin is secreted by the G cells in the antrum and the duodenum, and exists in the circulation in several forms, the major ones being G17 and G34, that is, the numbers of amino acids in each. They are occasionally referred to as 'small G' and 'big G' respectively. G17 is found in the stomach, and G34 mainly in the duodenum, and, in humans, in the circulation. The main physiological actions of gastrin are to release hydrochloric acid (HCl) from the parietal cells of the stomach, and to regulate growth of the gastric mucosa. The acidic gastric juice produced by gastrin excites pepsinogen secretion from the chief cells and secretin release from the S cell. Gastrin release is stimulated mainly by food, and to a lesser extent by free fatty acids, amino acids and peptides, but dietary sugars do not release gastrin. The hormone is also released following autonomic vagal stimulation. As an endocrine hormone, gastrin increases motor activity in the GIT, stimulates secretion of enzymes from the pancreas, relaxes the pyloric sphincter and increases lower oesophageal sphincter pressure.

Gastrin may be a neurotransmitter and/or neurohormone. The C-terminal tetrapeptide fragment of gastrin, identical to that of CCK, has been reported in the rat hypothalamus and pituitary portal blood.

Cholecystokinin (CCK). In humans, CCK is present predominantly as an octapeptide, although in the pig, at least four larger CCK-like peptides have been isolated. CCK-secreting cells (I-cells) occur mainly in the duodenum and the proximal jejunum. CCK has also been described in neurones innervating the distal intestine. CCK is present in the brain, being relatively abundant in the frontal cortex, the hypothalamus, the hippocampus and the amygdala. In the GIT, CCK is released in response to certain amino acids, particularly tryptophan and phenylalanine, lipids and free fatty acids.

In the GIT, CCK contracts the gall bladder (hence its name), and it stimulates the release of pancreatic enzymes. CCK stimulates glucagon release, as does VIP (see below). In older textbooks, CCK was called pancreozymin, but CCK and pancreozymin are one and the same thing. CCK enhances the action of secretin in stimulating bicarbonate release from the pancreas, and it delays gastric emptying. CCK, or a related peptide, may serve as a satiety hormone, since it reduces eating behaviour in humans and other animals, and it has been suggested that patients who suffer from bulimia nervosa, in which they eat obsessively, may have a deficiency of CCK secretion after eating.

Secretin. In humans, secretin is found predominantly in the granular S cells in the villi and crypts of the small intestinal mucosa. In the rat and pig, secretin has been found in the pituitary and pineal glands. Secretin is released in response to acidification of the contents of the duodenum, that is, the entry of gastric fluids. Secretin is not released above a pH of 4.5.

Its major action is to stimulate bicarbonate secretion from the pancreas, and it potentiates CCK-invoked release of pancreatic enzymes. Clearly, there is a negative-feedback relationship between secretin and bicarbonate which inhibits secretin release.

Vasointestinal peptide (VIP). Human VIP is a strongly basic polypeptide of 28 amino acids, belonging to the secretin family of peptides. The structure has been conserved, being identical in human, rat and pig. VIP is widely distributed throughout the body, but especially in the GIT, where it occurs throughout GIT length, from oesophagus to rectum. VIP-containing neurones are especially concentrated in the jejunum, ileum, colon, gall bladder wall, the sphincters and the pancreas. The factors which release VIP are not known with certainty, and there appear to be many. VIP release from cells is known to be modified by other neurones, which contain opioids (endogenous morphine-like peptides) and somatostatin as neurotransmitters. An important function of VIP within the gut may be to promote descending relaxation, as it is released only during relaxation.

Gastric inhibitory peptide (GIP) is a 42 amino acid polypeptide of the secretin family, present in the GIT at highest concentrations in the duodenum and jejunum. GIP release is stimulated by glucose, amino acids and free fatty acids, and release may also be modified by other hormones. An important action of GIP is to enhance insulin secretion from the pancreatic islet cells under conditions of hyperglycaemia. It is known that glucose taken orally is more potent in stimulating insulin release than when taken intravenously, and this may be explained by the stimulant effect of glucose on GIP release.

Gastrin releasing peptide (GRP), also called bombesin (when it was orginally isolated from frog skin), is a 27 amino acid (porcine) peptide present in the brain and GIT neurones. GRP, when introduced into rat brain, causes gastrin release from the G cell. GRP has been localized to nerve cells in the antral mucosa, and has been shown to produce a release of gastrin.

Enteroglucagon is the name given to an heterogeneous group of peptides within the gut. These are fragments of the proglucagon molecule, and include a peptide termed oxyntomodulin, and glicentin and GRPP (see page 82). The highest concentrations occur in the ileum and colon, and about 60–80% of the activity is accounted for by glicentin. The peptides are released by food in the gut, which is not the stimulus for glucagon release. The peptides are powerful inhibitors of gastric acid secretion from the parietal cells, and oxyntomodulin also stimulates liver glycogenolysis insulin release, although with less potency than glucagon.

Many other substances are released by the GIT, which appears to be the largest endocrine organ in the body; many more are reported as time goes by, and the reader is referred to the Further Reading section on page 103 for more information.

40 Endocrine hormones and energy metabolism

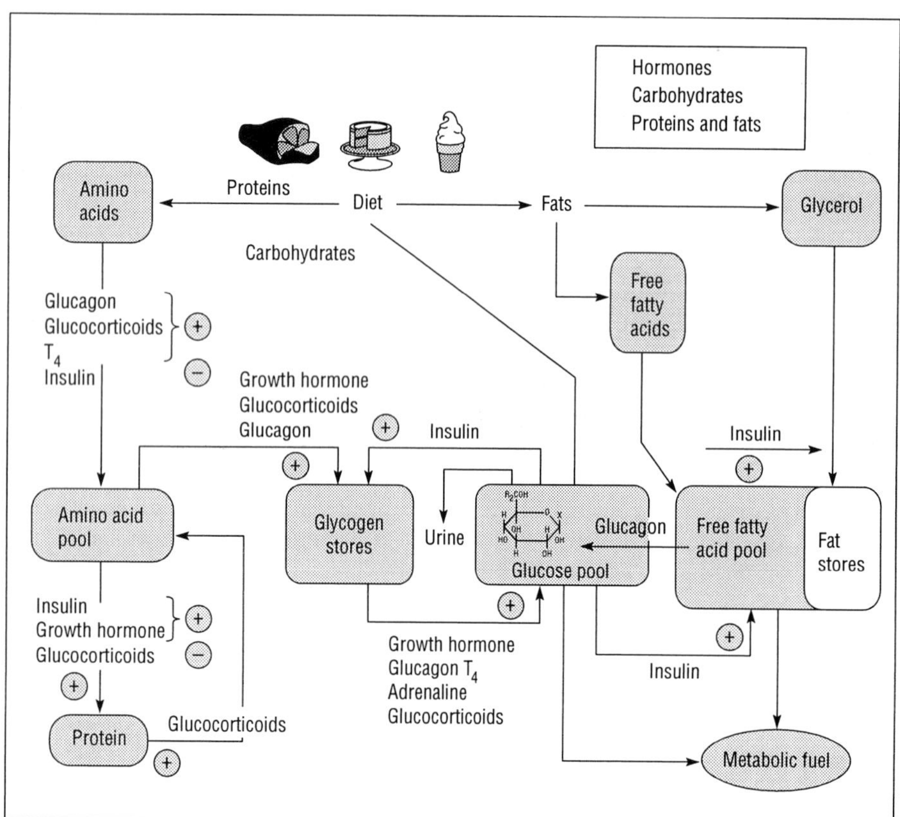

Fig. 40.1 Metabolism.

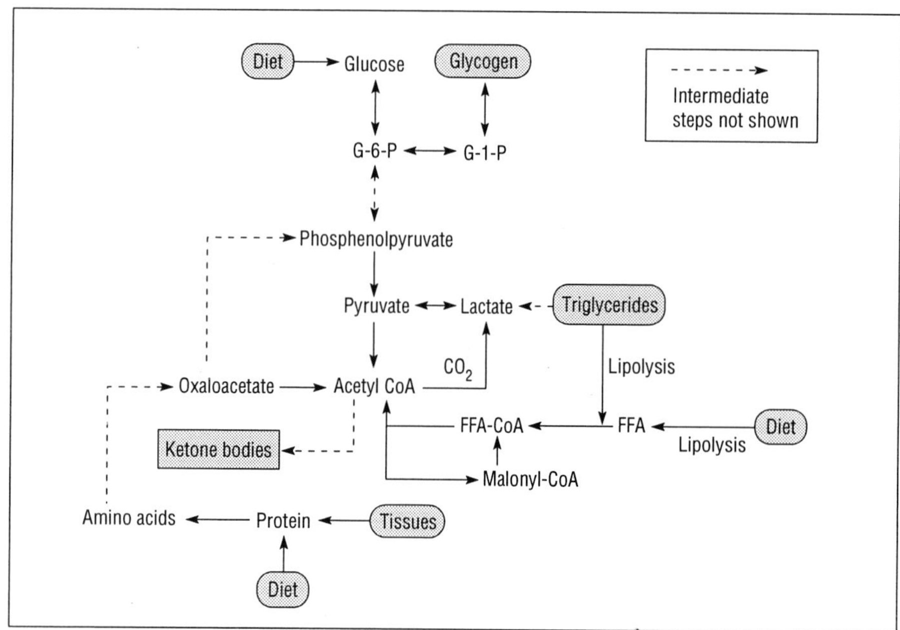

Fig. 40.2 Metabolism summary.

The endocrine control of energy metabolism is complex, but centres on the maintenance of an adequate supply of glucose for metabolism.

ENERGY STORES

Fats are the main energy stores in the body. Fats provide the most efficient means of storing energy in terms of KJ/g, and the body can store seemingly unlimited amounts of fat, a fact evident from the phenomenon of extreme obesity. Carbohydrate constitutes <1% of energy stores, and since tissues such as the brain are absolutely dependent on a constant supply of glucose, this must be supplied in the diet or by gluconeogenesis. Proteins contain about 20% of the body's energy stores, but since proteins have a structural and functional role, their integrity is defended, except in fasting, and these stores are therefore not readily available.

Circulating glucose can be considered as a *glucose pool*, which is in a dynamic state of equilibrium, balancing the inflow and outflow of glucose. The sources of inflow are the diet (carbohydrates) and hepatic glycogenolysis. The outflows are to the tissues, for glycogen synthesis, for energy use, or, if plasma concentrations reach a sufficient level, into the urine. This level is not usually reached in normal, healthy people.

Regulation of the glucose flows is through the action of endocrine hormones, these being adrenaline, growth hormone insulin, glucagon, glucocorticoids and thyroxine. Insulin is the only hormone with a hypoglycaemic action, whereas all the others are hyperglycaemic, since they stimulate glycogenolysis. Thus, falling blood glucose stimulates their release, while raised glucose stimulates insulin release, an example of dual negative-feedback control.

Integration of fat, carbohydrate and protein metabolism is essential for the effective control of the glucose pool. Two other pools are drawn upon for this, these being the free fatty acid (FFA) pool and the amino acid (AA) pool. The FFA pool comprises the balance between dietary FFA absorbed from the GIT, FFA released from adipose tissue after lipolysis, and FFA entering the metabolic process. Insulin drives FFA into storage as lipids, while glucagon, growth hormone and adrenaline stimulate lipolysis. The AA pool in the bloodstream comprises the balance between protein synthesis and the entry of amino acids into the gluconeogenic pathways. The term 'gluconeogenesis' literally means 'making new glucose'.

41 Endocrine regulation of calcium: I

ROLE OF CALCIUM (CA^{2+})

Calcium is essential for many physiological processes. It is required, for example, in bone growth, blood clotting, maintenance of the transmembrane potential, cell replication, stimulus-contraction and stimulus-secretion coupling, and in the second messenger process.

Circulating and extracellular calcium in adult humans is kept at a concentration of approximately 10 mg/dl. This equilibrium is achieved mainly in the kidney and the digestive tract, and by an ongoing exchange between the bone and extracellular fluid. About half the circulating ion is free and the rest is bound to plasma albumin. Circulating Ca^{2+} equilibrium is upset by protein abnormalities, acid–base disturbances, and by changes in the concentrations of plasma albumin. Bone provides the largest pool of Ca^{2+}, a smaller pool is provided by the soft tissues, and an even smaller pool by the extracellular fluid. Growing children are in a positive Ca^{2+} balance, and over the first 18 years postnatally, they will retain about 1 kg of calcium.

REGULATION OF CALCIUM

This is principally through three hormones: parathyroid hormone (PTH), from the parathyroid gland, which increases circulating Ca^{2+}; calcitonin from the parafollicular cells of the thyroid, which lowers Ca^{2+}; and 1,25-dihydroxy-vitamin D_3, a metabolite of vitamin D, which increases circulating Ca^{2+} ions.

The parathyroid glands are present in all terrestrial vertebrates. In humans, there are four parathyroid glands, consisting of adipocytes and chief cells, which contain the hormone. There are other cells, called oxyphil cells, which increase in number after puberty, and whose function is unknown. Removal of the parathyroid glands results in a fall in plasma Ca^{2+}, and convulsions and death.

Parathyroid hormone is also called parathormone and is abbreviated to PTH.

SYNTHESIS AND SECRETION

PTH is a polypeptide of 84 amino acids, cleaved from a pro-

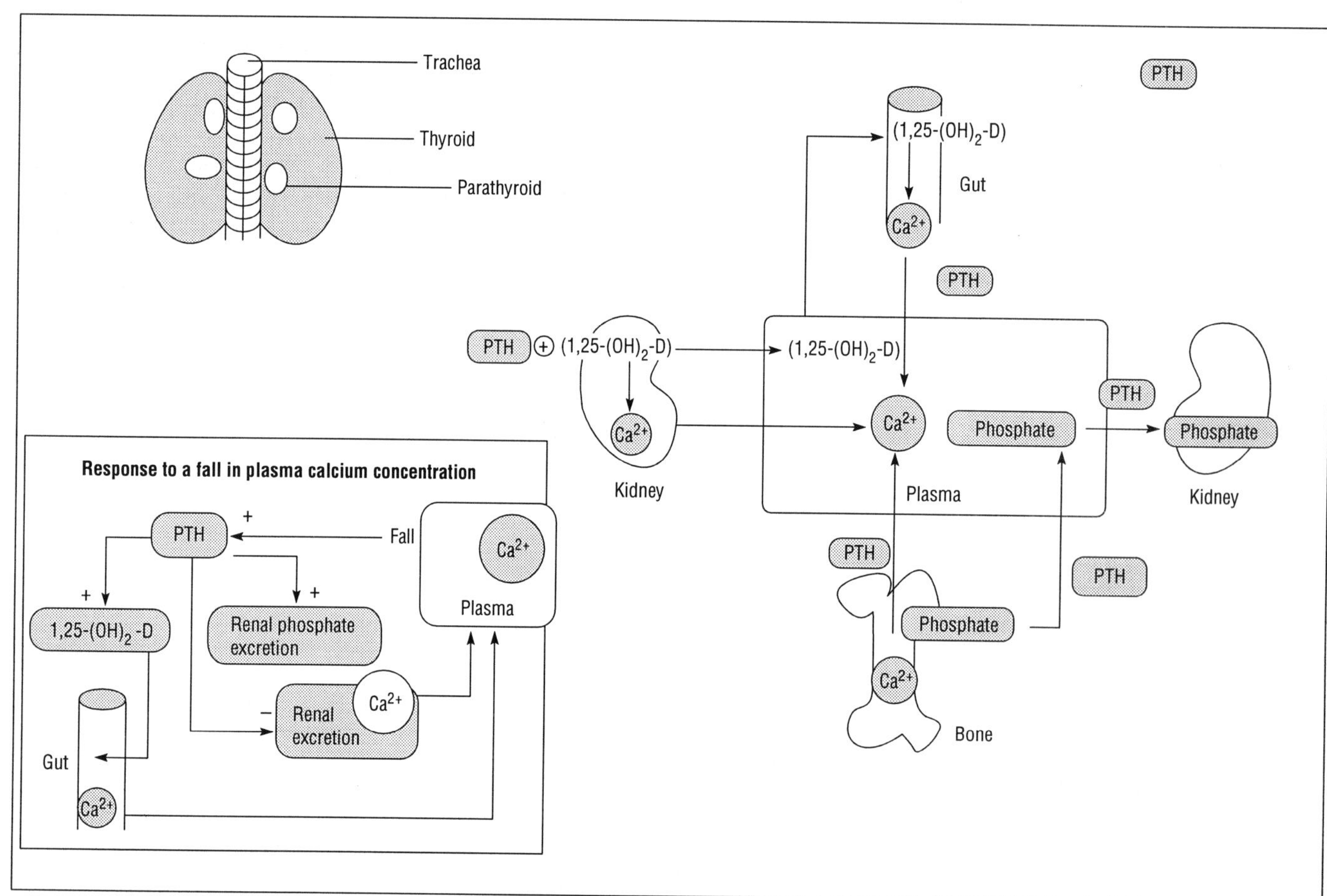

Fig. 41.1 Actions of parathyroid hormone.

PTH of 90 amino acids, which in turn is cleaved from a prepro-PTH of 115 amino acids. Cleavage of pro-PTH to PTH occurs about 15 minutes after arrival at the Golgi apparatus of pro-PTH, which is packaged in vesicles which are released by exocytosis. The PTH gene is localized to the short arm of chromosome 11.

Secretion is controlled by plasma Ca^{2+}. There is an inverse relationship between plasma Ca^{2+} and PTH. The parathyroid chief cells have recognition sites for Ca^{2+}, and the second messenger appears to be cAMP. PTH is cleaved in the circulation, the liver and the kidney, and one of the circulating fragments (1–34) retains biological activity.

PHYSIOLOGICAL ACTIONS OF PARATHYROID HORMONE

Bone. PTH acts on bone to liberate Ca^{2+}, orthophosphate, magnesium, citrate, hydroxyproline and osteocalcin, which forms 1–28% of all bone protein, and which has a high affinity for Ca^{2+}. PTH therefore has a resorptive effect on bone, which is probably direct on the osteoblasts, which then stimulate osteoclasts. Osteoblasts synthesize collagen, on which calcium phosphate precipitates as hydroxyapatite crystals. Bone is demineralized by the osteoclast cells, which release hyaluronic acid and acid phosphatase, which solubilize calcium phosphate.

Gastrointestinal tract. PTH stimulates the uptake of Ca^{2+} from the GIT, but this is an indirect action, exerted through the effects of PTH on vitamin D metabolism (see page 88).

Kidney. PTH enhances the urinary excretion of phosphate through a direct action on the proximal tubules of the kidney. This stimulates Ca^{2+} resorption of bone because it promotes Ca^{2+} ionization through the reduction in the $[Ca^{2+}] \times [PO_4^-]$ solubility product. In addition, PTH inhibits bicarbonate reabsorption, which produces a metabolic acidosis, which favours Ca^{2+} ionization, resulting in resorption of Ca^{2+} from bone, and dissociation of Ca^{2+} from plasma protein binding sites.

Other effects of parathyroid hormone. PTH dilates coronary and other vascular beds, possibly through a direct action on the smooth muscle of the arterioles.

PATHOPHYSIOLOGY OF PARATHYROID HORMONE

Assay of parathyroid hormone is usually indirect, through measurement of urinary and plasma cAMP. Urinary secretion of cAMP is reduced in conditions of hypercalcaemia of non-parathyroid origin, and increased in primary hyperparathyroidism. Radioimmunoassay (RIA) of PTH is difficult because of the various fragments in plasma, but an assay for PTH (1–84) is used, as well as one which uses an antiserum directed against a synthetic derivative of human or bovine PTH (53–84).

Primary hyperparathyroidism is caused either by a parathyroid adenoma or, more rarely, by a parathyroid carcinoma or through hereditary disease of the parathyroid gland. Patients present with the symptoms of hypercalcaemia, including mental confusion, headache, polyuria, polydipsia, calcified cornea, and renal and gallstone problems, including lithiasis (kidney and gall stones), due to deposition of insoluble phosphate salts, and pancreatitis (pancreas inflammation), which is associated with gallstones. There will be radiological evidence of bone resorption.

Ectopic hyperparathyroidism may be seen in patients with PTH-secreting tumours, and secondary hyperparathyroidism is associated with avitaminosis D, a lack of vitamin D, resulting in reduced Ca^{2+} absorption from the GIT, which in turn stimulates PTH release. Treatment is by infusing Ca^{2+}.

Hypoparathyroidism or PTH deficiency leads to hypocalcaemia. This produces central effects, such as convulsions and psychotic states. Peripheral symptoms include tetany, laryngiospasm, degenerative changes in teeth, fingernails, and in cataract. The patient is hypocalcinaemic and has hyperphosphataemia. The causes of hypoparathyroidism may be through mechanical injury to the neck, as in a motor car accident, and, more rarely, hereditary absence of the glands, or destruction by a tumour. Treatment is with oral Ca^{2+} plus calcitriol (1,25-dihydroxy-vitamin D_3).

42 Endocrine regulation of calcium: II

CALCITONIN

Calcitonin is a hypocalcaemic polypeptide hormone. In mammals, it is synthesized and secreted in parafollicular (C) cells in the thyroid gland. C cells have been found in much lower density in the parathyroid glands and in the thymus. In fish and birds, calcitonin is synthesized within a specific organ, the ultimobranchial body. The ultimobranchial bodies do develop in mammals during fetal life, but eventually disappear. It is thought that the C cells evolved before the parathyroids, to help sea-dwelling animals to cope with the relatively high concentrations of calcium (Ca^{2+}) in sea water.

Biosynthesis and secretion. Calcitonin (CT) is synthesized in C (clear) cells from a larger 136 amino acid precurser, called calcitonin precursor, or prohormone, from which CT is cleaved, together with two other peptides of unknown function. The gene which encodes CT has been characterized, and is expressed not only in the C cells of the thyroid, but also in the brain. In neural tissue, however, the gene expresses not CT but another peptide, the calcitonin gene-related peptide (CGRP). This is therefore an example of tissue-determining expression of a common gene. The function of CRGP has not been elucidated. The gene occurs on the short arm of chromosome 11, probably near the insulin gene.

At normal plasma Ca^{2+} levels, CT release is low, but a rise in Ca^{2+} causes a rapid (threefold) rise in CT concentrations. Even if a small amount of Ca^{2+}, which is insufficient to raise plasma concentrations of the ion in plasma, reaches the gastrointestinal tract (GIT), CT is released. It is therefore thought that other GIT factors, for example, gastrin and/or cholecystokinin, (CCK) may trigger CT secretion. The sensitivity of the CT-release mechanism is sexually differentiated, being greater in males, and the responsiveness of the CT release mechanism declines with ageing. The half-life of CT in plasma is less than 15 minutes, and it may be degraded and excreted principally by the kidney.

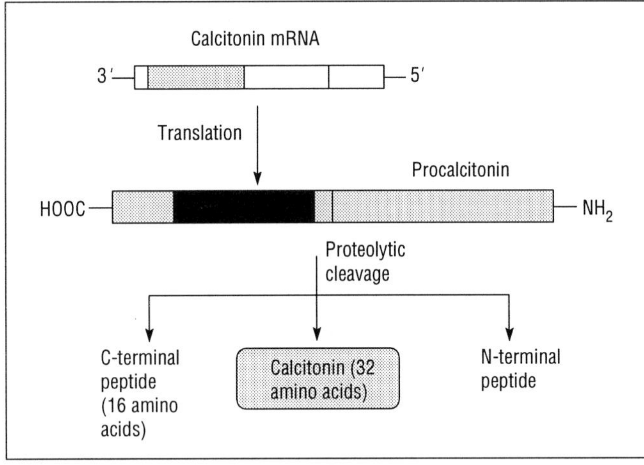

Fig. 42.1 Calcitonin synthesis.

Physiological actions of calcitonin. In humans, calcitonin is not as important as is PTH in the regulation of Ca^{2+} metabolism. The two main target organs for CT are *bone* and *kidney*. In bone, CT is a potent inhibitor of resorption, both *in vivo* and *in vitro*, although CT has no effects on bone formation. There is an inhibition of calcium resorption by the osteoclasts within 20 minutes of administration of a dose of CT. CT may be particularly important during periods of threatened increased Ca^{2+} loss, such as occurs during pregnancy and lactation.

In the kidney, CT is concentrated in the renal cortex. Membranes of the tubule cells possess specific CT receptors, and the

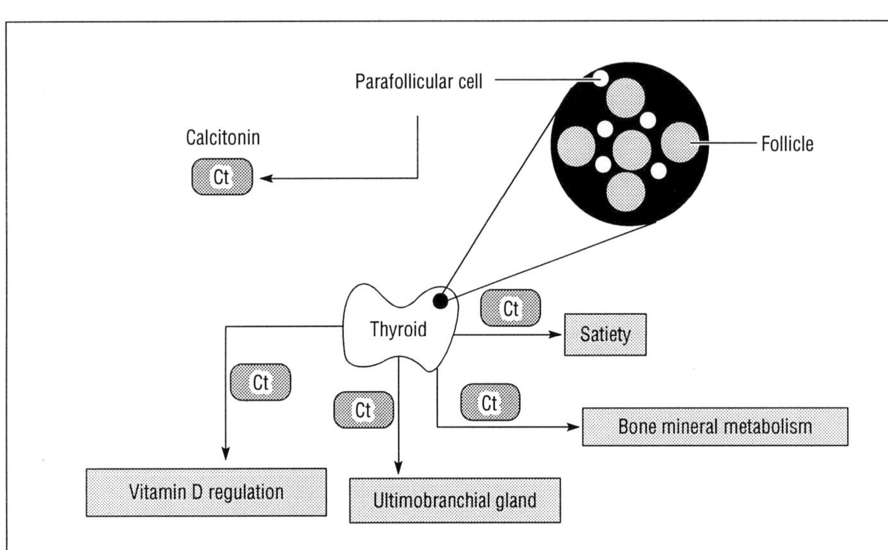

Fig. 42.2 Role of calcitonin.

second messenger may be adenylate cyclase, although administration of CT does not appear to alter cellular levels of cAMP. In the kidney, CT increases the excretion of Ca^{2+}, Na^{+} and K^{+}, and reduces excretion of Mg^{2+}.

CT may be important in the regulation of postprandial feeding, to prevent food-induced hypercalcaemia. CT may also be a satiety hormone. In humans, injection of CT is followed by a significant fall in body weight within 36 hours, and CT inhibits feeding behaviour in rhesus monkeys and rats. The hormone is particularly potent when administered directly to the brain, suggesting that it may have a central role.

CT affects *vitamin D* metabolism by lowering plasma Ca^{2+}, resulting in the release of PTH, which in turn promotes the production and secretion of vitamin D metabolites in the kidney.

Calcitonin pathophysiology. Many thyroid tumours produce CT, or hypercalcitonaemia may be hereditary through an autosomal dominant trait. Elevated CT has been observed in patients with pancreatitis and in acute hepatitis. Loss of CT from the circulation may result from surgical or isotopic destruction of the thyroid.

CT is used in the treatment of hypercalcaemia, most commonly in children suffering from hyperparathyroidism, bone metastasis, hypercalcaemia of unknown origin (idiopathic), and in cases of vitamin D intoxication. Its principal use is in the treatment of Paget's disease, a chronic bone disease occurring mainly in the elderly, which affects the skull, backbone, pelvis and the long bones. CT abolishes the pain associated with the disease and improves the skeletal abnormalities.

43 Endocrine regulation of calcium: III

VITAMIN D

Vitamins are not generally considered to be hormones, but organic dietary factors essential for healthy life. The term 'vitamin' is perhaps a misnomer therefore for the substances called vitamin D. The name actually refers to two steroid-like chemicals, namely *ergocalciferol* and *cholecalciferol*, which prevent or cure rickets. Rickets is a disease of children, when the bones do not harden and become malformed due to an insufficiency of calcium (Ca^{2+}) without which the bones do not become rigid, and bend.

Osteomalacia is the softening of bones in adults who suffer from a deficiency of vitamin D in the diet, or of sunlight, or both. It is most common in the Middle and Far East, in women who lose calcium through pregnancy, and especially in those societies where much of the body is covered in dark clothing.

SYNTHESIS

The active form of vitamin D is 1-alpha, 25-dihydroxyvitamin D_3 (25-$(OH)_2$-D_3). Ultraviolet irradiation in sunlight photo-isomerizes a cholesterol precursor, 7-dehydrocholesterol, which converts it to pre-vitamin D, which then undergoes a thermal isomerization to cholecalciferol (vitamin D_3). Cholecalciferol binds in the dermis to a binding protein, which transports it in the plasma, and it is converted in the liver to 25-hydroxyvitamin D_3 (25-OH-D_3). This metabolite circulates, and in the kidney it is converted into the active metabolite 1-alpha-$(OH)_2$-D_3.

REGULATION OF METABOLISM

The regulation of vitamin D_3 metabolism is bound up with that of parathyroid hormone (PTH). PTH secretion from the parathyroid glands is stimulated by hypocalcaemia. PTH stimulates the kidney cortex mitochondrial enzyme 1-alpha-hydroxylase, which is also stimulated by low concentrations of phosphate. The 1-alpha-$(OH)_2$-D_3 thus formed enters the circulation and promotes Ca^{2+} resorption from bone; Ca^{2+} absorption from the gastrointestinal tract (GIT); stimulates the reabsorption of Ca^{2+} from the kidney; and the excretion of phosphate. The hypercalcaemia created inhibits further production of PTH, which in turn limits the synthesis of 1-alpha-$(OH)_2$-D_3. The active metabolite is inactivated by conversion to 24,25-$(OH)_2$-D_3. 1-alpha-$(OH)_2$-D_3 may also feed back to the parathyroid glands to inhibit the release of PTH. The glands do possess receptors for 1-alpha-$(OH)_2$-D_3.

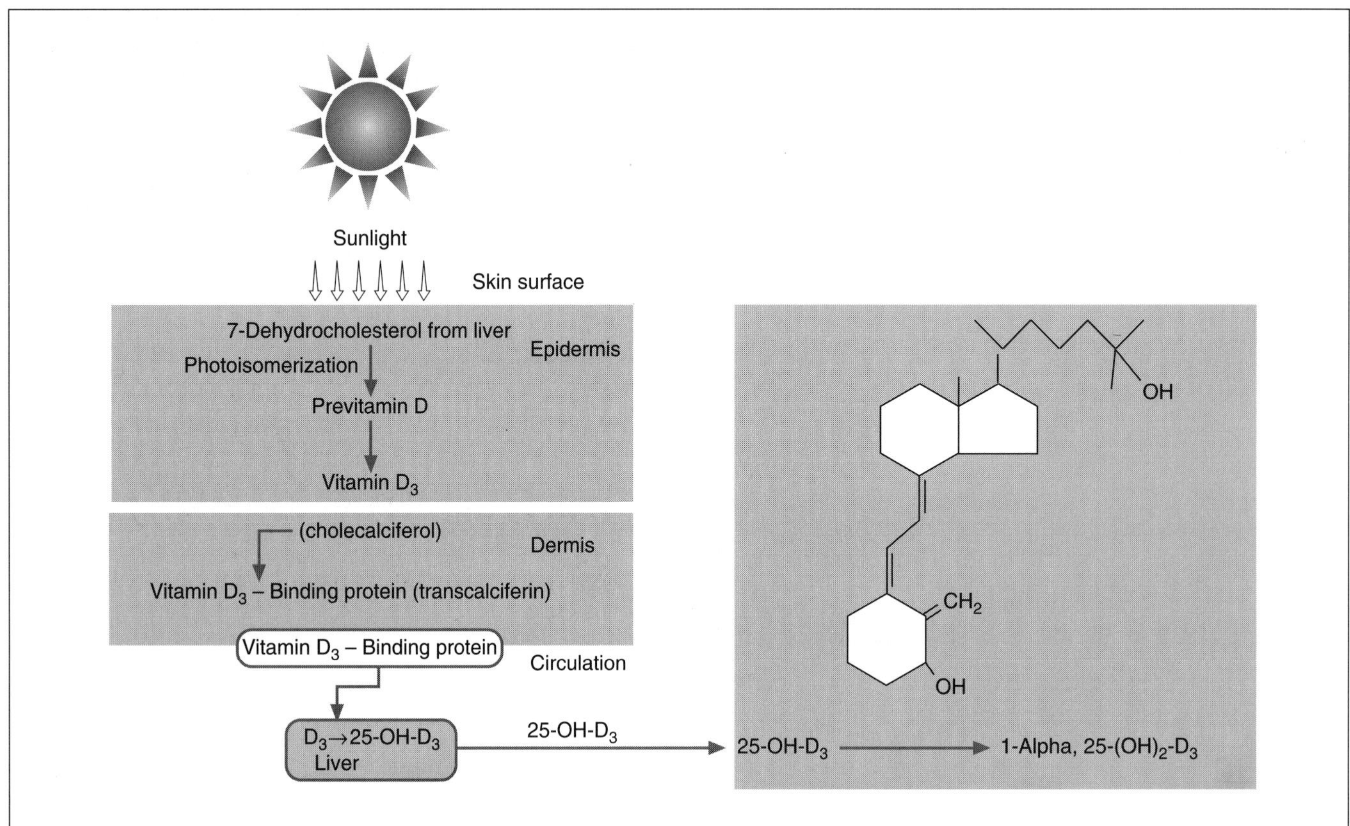

Fig. 43.1 Synthesis of vitamin D.

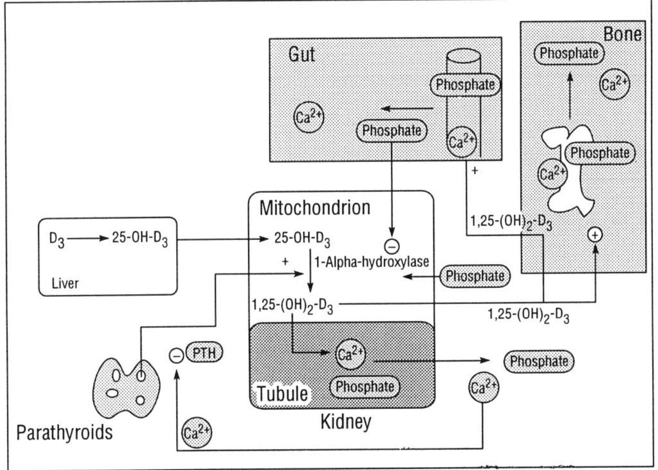

Fig. 43.2 Regulation of vitamin D.

MECHANISM OF ACTION

The 1-alpha-$(OH)_2$-D_3 receptor belongs to a superfamily of nuclear hormone receptors, which bind to their ligand and alter transcription (see page 15). The hormone travels in the bloodstream in equilibrium between bound and free forms. The latter form is freely able to enter cells, due to its lipophilic nature. The plasma 1-alpha-$(OH)_2$-D_3-binding protein (DBP) recognizes the hormone specifically. 1-alpha-$(OH)_2$-D_3 binds to the nuclear receptor; the complex binds to specific hormone response elements on the target gene upstream of transcriptional activation sites, and new mRNA and protein synthesis result. New proteins synthesized include osteocalcin, an important bone protein, whose synthesis is suppressed by glucocorticoids. In the GIT, a calcium-binding transport protein (CaBP) is synthesized in response to the hormone–receptor activation of the genome.

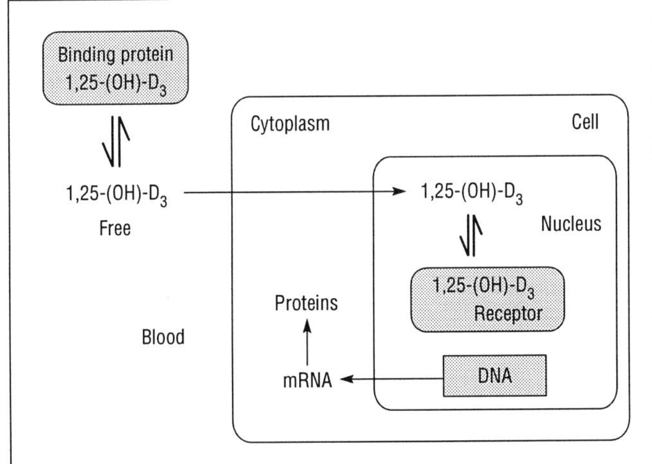

Fig. 43.3 Mechanism of action of vitamin D.

PHYSIOLOGICAL ACTIONS OF VITAMIN D

Bone. Vitamin D stimulates resorption of Ca^{2+} from bone as part of its function to maintain adequate circulating concentrations of the ion. It also stimulates osteocalcin synthesis.

Gastrointestinal tract. 1-alpha-$(OH)_2$-D_3 stimulates Ca^{2+} and phosphate absorption from the gut through an active transport process. The hormone promotes the synthesis of calcium transport by enhancing synthesis of the cytosolic calcium-binding protein CaBP, which transports Ca^{2+} from the mucosal to the serosal cells of the gut.

Kidney. 1-alpha-$(OH)_2$-D_3 may stimulate reabsorption of Ca^{2+} into the tubule cells while promoting the excretion of phosphate. The tubule cells do possess receptors for vitamin D and CaBP.

Muscle. Muscle cells have vitamin D receptors, and the hormone may mediate muscle contraction through effects on the calcium fluxes, and on consequent adenosine triphosphate (ATP) synthesis.

Pregnancy. During pregnancy, there is increased Ca^{2+} absorption from the GIT, and elevated circulating concentrations of 1-alpha-$(OH)_2$-D_3, DBP, calcitonin and PTH. During the last 6 months prior to birth, Ca^{2+} and phosphorus accumulate in the fetus. The placenta synthesizes 1-alpha-$(OH)_2$-D_3, as does the fetal kidney and bone. Nevertheless, the fetus still requires maternal vitamin D.

Other roles. Vitamin D may be involved in the maturation and proliferation of cells of the immune system, for example, of the haematopoietic stem cells, and in the function of mature B and T cells.

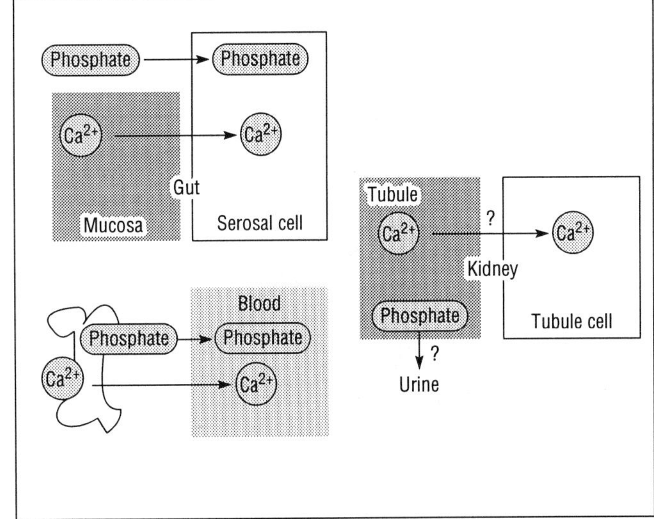

Fig. 43.4 Physiological actions of vitamin D.

44 Growth hormones: I

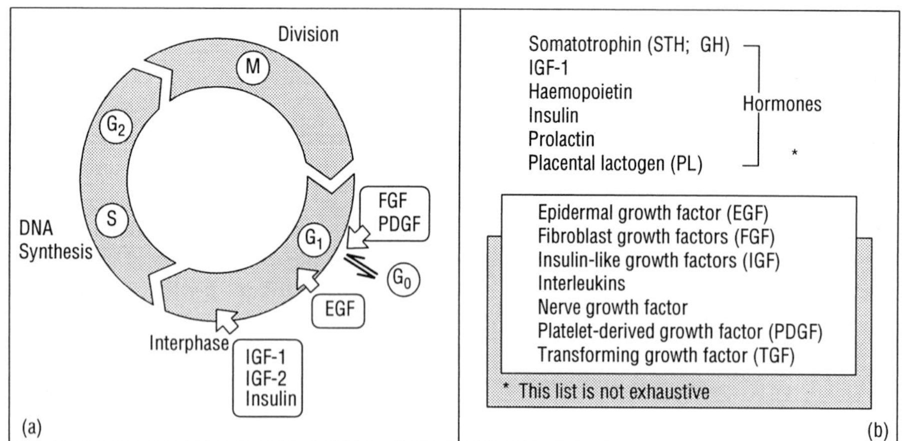

Fig. 44.1 (a) The cell cycle; (b) growth hormones and factors.

CELLULAR GROWTH AND PROLIFERATION

Cell differentiation and organ development depend on the action of autocrine, paracrine and endocrine hormones. A large number of growth factors which promote cellular proliferation, have been discovered. Furthermore, hormones such as insulin and prolactin are growth hormones, in addition to their classically accepted roles in glucose metabolism, pregnancy and lactation respectively.

The cell cycle. Dividing cells pass through stages which are dependent on the action of growth factors and hormones. The growth phase is G_1; this phase prepares the cell for the synthetic phase S, during which the DNA becomes duplicated. Thereafter, the cell splits into two daughter cells in the M phase. The new cells may remain in G_0 and never divide again (e.g. neurones, muscle cells), or they may enter G_1 to repeat the cycle. Tumour cells may remain in G_0 before re-entering G_1. The growth factors and hormones act at specific phases of the cell cycle.

Insulin-like growth factor (IGF). IGF-1 and IGF-2 together are called the *somatomedins*, because they mediate the actions of somatotrophin (STH). Their molecular weight is about 7.6 kDa, and they share 62% sequence homology. IGF is the abbreviated form of insulin-like growth factor, so-called because the somatomedins cross-react in some radioimmunoassays for insulin, and because they have structures similar to that of pro-insulin. The somatomedins are synthesized mainly in the liver, although fibroblasts and pituitary and other cell types synthesize them. Both IGF-1 and 2 bind to insulin receptors, and the structure of the insulin receptor is similar to that of the IGF receptors.

The actions of somatotrophic hormone (STH) on growth are mediated mainly by IGF-1. STH causes the release of IGF-1 from the liver. The IGFs circulate in plasma tightly bound to proteins, which protect them from proteolysis, and thus maintain their concentrations in plasma. Although the physiological function of IGF-2 is unknown, it is at least three times more abundant in the circulation of the adult human than IGF-1. Plasma levels of both somatomedins remain fairly constant in the healthy adult, but rise sharply during postnatal development, reaching a peak between 12 and 17 years, and fall thereafter. Both are powerful mitogens. IGF-1 is a proliferator of already differentiated cells, a process called clonal expansion.

Insulin. Apart from its important role in the control of carbohydrate metabolism, insulin is also a growth hormone, since diabetic children fail to grow normally even with normal plasma levels of STH. Without insulin, protein catabolism is enhanced, which works to inhibit growth, and amino acid uptake into muscle is inhibited, as is the process of translation of mRNA by the ribosomes.

Placental lactogen (PL) is a placental hormone, also called somatomammatrophin. Many of the actions of PL are similar to those of prolactin. PL promotes the incorporation of sulphur into cartilege, growth and the synthesis of milk protein. PL may play a physiological role in the development of the mammary glands, in preparation for the action of prolactin after parturition. PL antagonizes the actions of insulin, and promotes amino acid and glucose utilization in the fetus. During the second trimester of pregnancy, PL may take over the role of chorionic gonadotrophin, the levels of which begin to decline.

Prolactin (PRL) promotes the synthesis of milk. Together with adrenal steroids and oestrogens, PRL stimulates growth of the mammary duct system and, together with the gonadotrophins, growth of the ovaries and testes. PRL stimulates the production of a liver peptide, tentatively called synlactin, which possibly synergizes with PRL in its target organs. The secretion of prolactin is controlled by the hypothalamus.

Nerve growth factor (NGF) is a peptide similar in structure to pro-insulin. It is secreted in large amounts by the mouse submandibular glands, under the control of tri-iodothyronine, thyroxine and testosterone, and is therefore present in much larger quantities in the saliva of the male. NGF may play a role in fighting, since it is released into the bloodstream in huge amounts when male mice fight each other.

The peptide derived its name from its growth actions on peripheral postganglionic nerves, and on the growth of the nervous system of the developing chick embryo. Injection of NGF antiserum into the developing embryo causes widespread damage to the sympathetic division of the autonomic nervous system. NGF induces neurite growth and plays a role in the guidance of growing sympathetic fibres to the organs they will ultimately innervate. Cells in the path of the growing axon synthesize and release NGF. In the brain, NGF may have a role in maintaining memory, since it restores learning and memory to rats with brain lesions, which suggests that NGF may be useful in Alzheimer's disease.

Epidermal growth factor (EGF) is a 53 amino acid peptide, isolated from the mouse salivary gland, where it is associated with an EGF-binding protein. EGF is released by alpha-adrenergic agonists, suggesting that release is under autonomic control. In the embryo and neonatal mouse, EGF promotes proliferation of the cells of the epidermis, the opening of the eyelids and the eruption of teeth. EGF promotes the maturation of the epithelium of the developing lungs, the keratinization of the skin and the phosphorylation of proteins. EGF is present in breast milk as a mitogenic factor.

EGF is similar in structure to a peptide called *urogastrone*, which was identified in the urine of pregnant women who enjoyed a remission from gastric ulcers during their pregnancy. Urogastrone is a gastrointestinal tract (GIT) peptide which inhibits gastric secretion in the gastric mucosa. Human urogastrone may be the human equivalent of EGF.

Transforming growth factors (TGF). TGF-alpha and TGF-beta are peptides which cause the growth of fibroblast cells. TGF-alpha is a 50 amino acid peptide, structurally similar to EGF. It binds to the EGF receptor and shares many of the actions of EGF. TGF-alpha itself exists in five forms (TGF-alpha-1–TGF-alpha-5).

TGF-beta exists in at least five forms, TGF-beta-1–5, and was originally discovered in platelets. It is present in most cells, especially in bone matrix, which contains relatively large amounts of the peptide. In bone, TGF-beta may be important in chondrocyte, osteoblast and osteoclast differentiation and growth.

TGF-beta can be stimulatory or inhibitory to the growth of non-endothelial cells, depending on the presence or absence of other factors. It does not bind to the EGF receptor. It may be inhibitory or stimulatory to organ and tumour growth, and modulates the action of other growth factors, including that of EGF. TGF-beta has structural homology with the Müllerian regression factor and inhibin.

The fibroblast growth factor (FGF) family includes acidic (aFGF), basic (bFGF), keratinocyte and other polypeptide growth factors which share several properties, including substantial sequence homology, angiogenesis promotion, heparin binding and mitogenic action in several different cell types. They are also called heparin-binding growth factors (HBGF). Binding to heparin stabilizes the factors and enhances their biological activities. They have been isolated from serum and from bone, brain, adrenal cortex, ovary and retina. Both a and b forms have a molecular weight of about 17 kDa and 55% sequence homology.

Angiogenesis is the formation, proliferation and migration of new blood vessels, a process essential in health for growth, wound healing and revascularization of diseased heart and brain tissue, and in disease for the growth of both benign and malignant tumours. Little is known of the physiological significance of the FGFs, although bFGF may have a role in very early embryonic differentiation and growth. BFGF has been very highly conserved throughout evolution, being present in all vertebrates, including fish. The FGFs may provide a means of regenerating damaged tissue and promoting healing.

Platelet-derived growth factor (PDGF) is synthesized and stored in blood platelets, and released when platelets are activated during blood vessel injury. Other tissues synthesize and store PDGF. The peptide is a heterodimer of molecular weight of 30 kDa, consisting of A and B chains, and forms part of a larger family, depending on the nature of the dimerization of the two chains. The family consists of PDGF (AA), (AB), and (BB). AB is the predominant form present in platelets. There are two different receptors for PDGF, one which recognizes all the heterodimers, and one which recognizes only BB.

PDGF is a powerful cell growth promoter *in vitro*, has strong chemotactic properties, and appears to have a role in inflammation and tumour and cell growth.

Erythropoietin (EP) is erythrocyte-stimulating factor, produced in the kidneys, which travels to the bone marrow to stimulate production of mature red blood cells. The liver can maintain a low level of EP production in patients with kidney damage.

In plasma, EP is a protein of molecular weight of about 46 kDa, although in urine EP size is halved, suggesting that the protein is a dimer. EP has a half-life of 5 hours, while its effects are not manifested for at least 36 hours, a time sequence consistent with the probability that EP generates a sequence of haemopoietic events which are not dependent on its continuous presence for completion. EP stimulates the production of erythrocyte precursor cells, by causing the production of a cytoplasmic protein which interacts with the genome to initiate transcription, and all else follows independently of the presence of EP.

The interleukins are a family of at least eight proteins, gaining their name because they were originally derived from leukocytes. They are examples of the cytokines, a group of soluble proteins which act as intercellular communicators. IL-1 is produced by activated macrophages, and stimulates IL-2 production by T cells and proliferation and differentiation of B cells. IL-2 is produced by T cells activated during an immune response. IL-6 is interferon-beta, which is synthesized by fibroblasts and some tumour cells. It increases immunoglobulin synthesis, and has antiviral activity.

45 Growth hormones: II

SOMATOTROPHIN (STH; GROWTH HORMONE: GH)

STH is required for normal growth; without it, the individual becomes a dwarf. Oversecretion, on the other hand, will stimulate abnormal growth, and giantism results, illustrating the potential for the body to grow beyond (presumably) genetically determined limits.

Chemistry and synthesis. STH is synthesized in the somatotroph cells in the anterior pituitary gland. STH is a member of a family of polypeptide hormones, including *prolactin (PRL)* and *placental lactogen (PL)*. STH is a single chain 191 amino acid polypeptide, and has a high structural homology with PL and PRL. All three are derived from a common precursor, even though each hormone has its own gene. They share a common ancestral gene from which the STH/PL gene diverged about

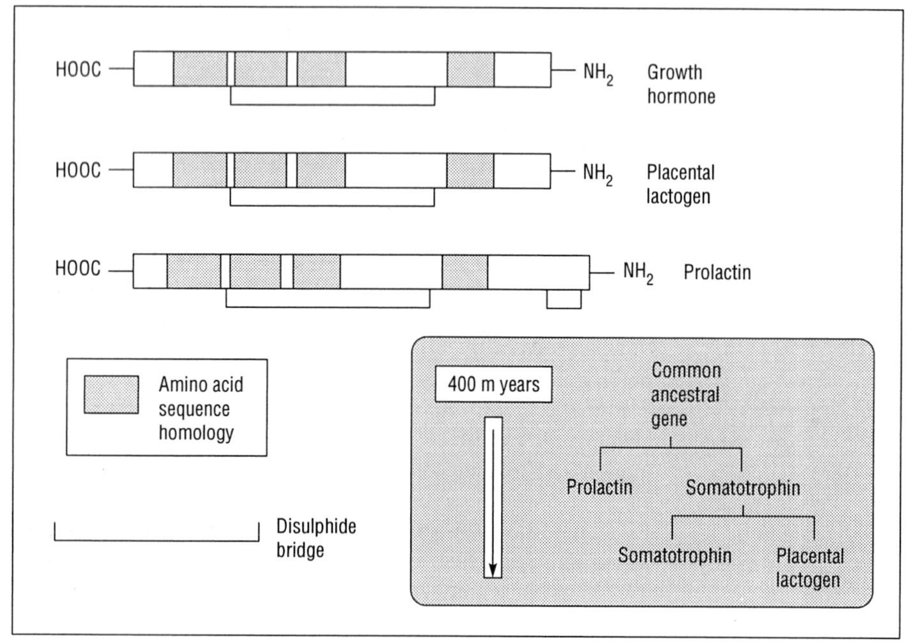

Fig. 45.1 Polypeptide hormone family (inset: evolution).

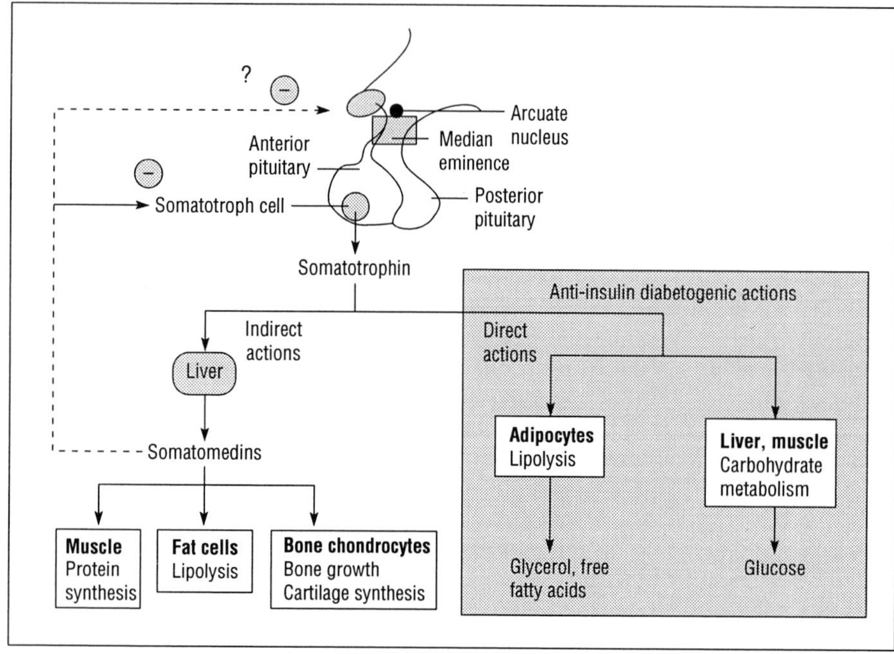

Fig. 45.2 Somatotrophin actions.

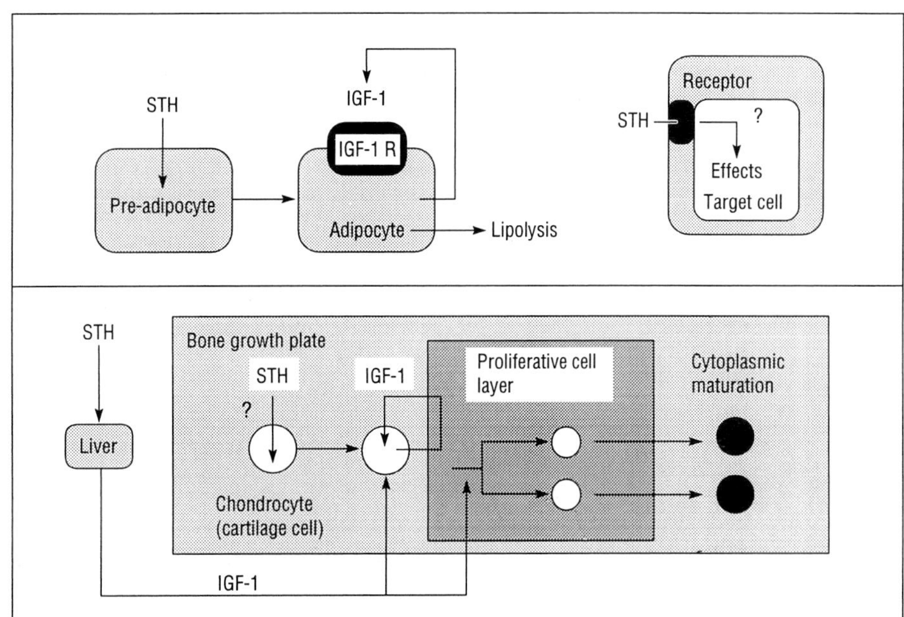

Fig. 45.3 Somatotrophin mechanism of action.

400 million years ago, and divergence of STH and PL genes occurred about 85–100 million years ago. The STH and PL genes exit as multiple copies on chromosome 17, and the PRL gene is a single copy on chromosome 6. Mouse fibroblasts synthesize a peptide called proliferin, which has significant structural homology with STH, PRL and PL, suggesting that this family may be larger than originally appreciated. STH and PRL exist in pituitary and plasma in more than one form, that is, they show structural heterogeneity.

Effects of somatotrophin. The most dramatic effect of STH is on muscle and skeletal bone growth. The effects may be conveniently divided into direct and indirect actions.

Indirect actions of somatotrophin. STH acts in the liver to stimulate the synthesis and secretion of the peptide insulin-like growth factor (IGF)-1.

In *bone*, STH appears to stimulate local production of IGF-1 in proliferative chondrocytes, apart from the production of IGF-1 in liver. The factor then stimulates bone growth. In *fat cells*, the factor stimulates lipolysis and in *muscle*, it stimulates protein synthesis.

The direct actions of STH have been termed diabetogenic, since the hormone's actions oppose those of insulin, being lipolytic in fat and gluconeogenic in muscle.

The mechanism of action of STH is largely unknown, except that it has a specific receptor on the membrane of the target cell. No changes in cAMP, phosphoinositol (the PLC/IP_3 system), nor in the activity of any tyrosine kinase enzyme, in response to STH, have been reported.

46 Growth hormones: III

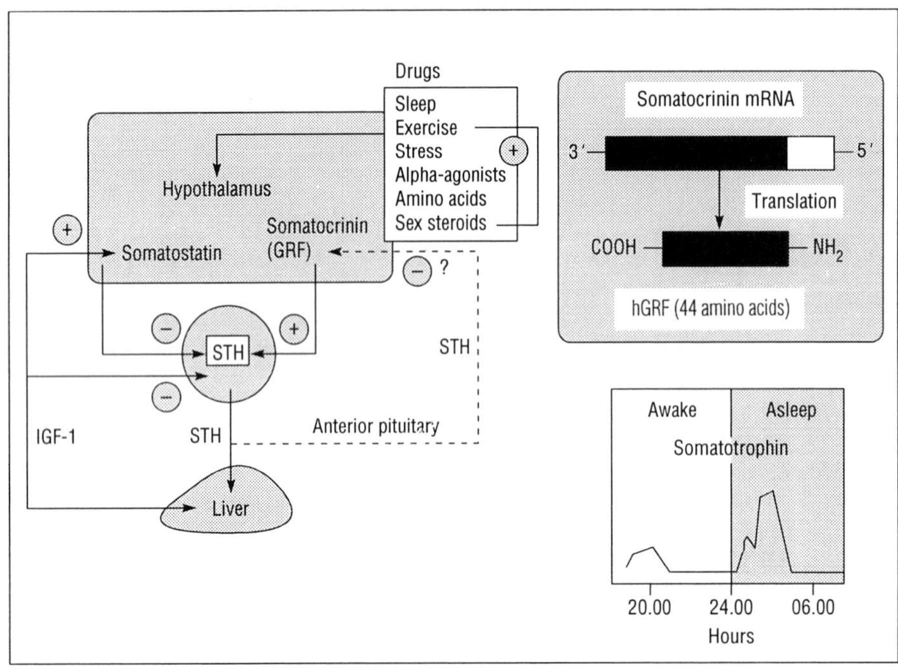

Fig. 46.1 Regulation of somatotrophin secretion.

REGULATION OF SOMATOTROPHIN SECRETION

Somatotrophin (STH) secretion is regulated primarily by the hypothalamus, which produces an STH-releasing hormone, best known as growth hormone-releasing hormone (GRH), and also referred to as *somatocrinin*.

GRH in humans is a 44 amino acid peptide, which is released into the portal system and binds to specific receptors on anterior pituitary somatotrophs, to stimulate STH release. The second messenger activated by GRH is cAMP, although the IP_3 system may also be activated. The hypothalamus also produces an inhibitory hormone called *somatostatin*, which inhibits STH release from somatotrophs. Somatostatin is a 14 amino acid peptide, which also exists in the hypothalamus in a 28 amino acid form. Both are active in inhibiting STH secretion, which they do by inhibiting cAMP production. Both GRH and somatostatin have been localized to the arcuate nucleus (see page 22). Several other factors affect STH release.

The physiological feedback control of STH release is mediated by insulin-like growth factor (IGF-1), which stimulates somatostatin secretion from the hypothalamus. IGF-1 also inhibits STH secretion directly.

STH secretion is episodic, peaking twice during the day, and rising in sleep, during the first hour, in both children and young adults.

PATHOPHYSIOLOGY OF SOMATOTROPHIN SECRETION

Deficiency of STH secretion. Deficiency of STH in growing children produces dwarfism.

Laron dwarfism is familial, transmitted as an autosomal recessive, and is especially prevalent in families in the Middle East. It is also termed idiopathic dwarfism. It is characterized by insensitivity of the liver to STH. The somatotroph produces normal STH, but circulating somatomedin concentrations are low.

In Laron dwarfism, there is a deficiency of STH receptors on circulating STH-binding proteins. This may reflect a problem with the STH-receptor interaction in the liver. African pygmies have normal STH plasma concentrations, but low IGF-1, presumably due to an inability to synthesize sufficient quantities of IGF-1. Some patients with dwarfism exhibit an inability to respond to IGF-1.

In *primary pituitary dwarfism*, STH deficiency may be genetic, or caused by tumours, or through the production of a form of STH which does not stimulate IGF-1 secretion from the liver, even though the STH reacts normally with antisera used in radioimmunoassay (RIA) for the hormone. The disease is associated with an increased overall mortality rate, due to cardiovascular disease.

Hypothalamic dwarfism is a variant on the pituitary form, in that no STH can be released, since no GRH is released into the portal circulation. This may result from an hypothalamic injury or from asphyxia during birth, or from infection or tumour growth.

Treatment. Human STH, known as human growth hormone, or hGH, has been in use therapeutically for over 30 years, although supply was restricted as it had to be extracted from human pituitaries. Nowadays hGH is synthesized using recombinant DNA techniques, which obviates the hazards inherent in using human-derived material, which carries with it the danger of infection. The main use of hGH is in the treatment of growth retardation in children. The use of GRH is also considered feasible in some quarters.

Excess somatotrophin secretion. Excess secretion of STH results in *acromegaly* in adults and *gigantism* in children. The usual source of excess STH secretion is a pituitary adenoma. Rarely, ectopic STH-producing tumours do occur. Acromegaly results in a coarsening of facial features and of the soft tissues of the hands and feet. Exaggerated growth of the mandible (lower jaw) occurs, resulting in a characteristic facial configuration. There is hypertrophy of connective tissue of the kidney, heart and liver, and the patient's glucose tolerance is lowered by up to 50%, resulting in diabetes in about 10% of patients with acromegaly. When diagnosing acromegaly, it is best to measure both STH and IGF-1 in the plasma of patients, especially when STH values are near-normal.

Treatment is to remove the source of excess STH and limit the secondary complications such as diabetes, progression of rheumatism and cardiovascular disease. Untreated acromegalic patients have approximately double the death rate of healthy individuals. Surgery may be resorted to in order to remove the pituitary (hypophysectomy). The pituitary may be irradiated. Some drugs are prescribed, notably bromocriptine, a dopamine agonist which lowers the secretion of STH and prolactin.

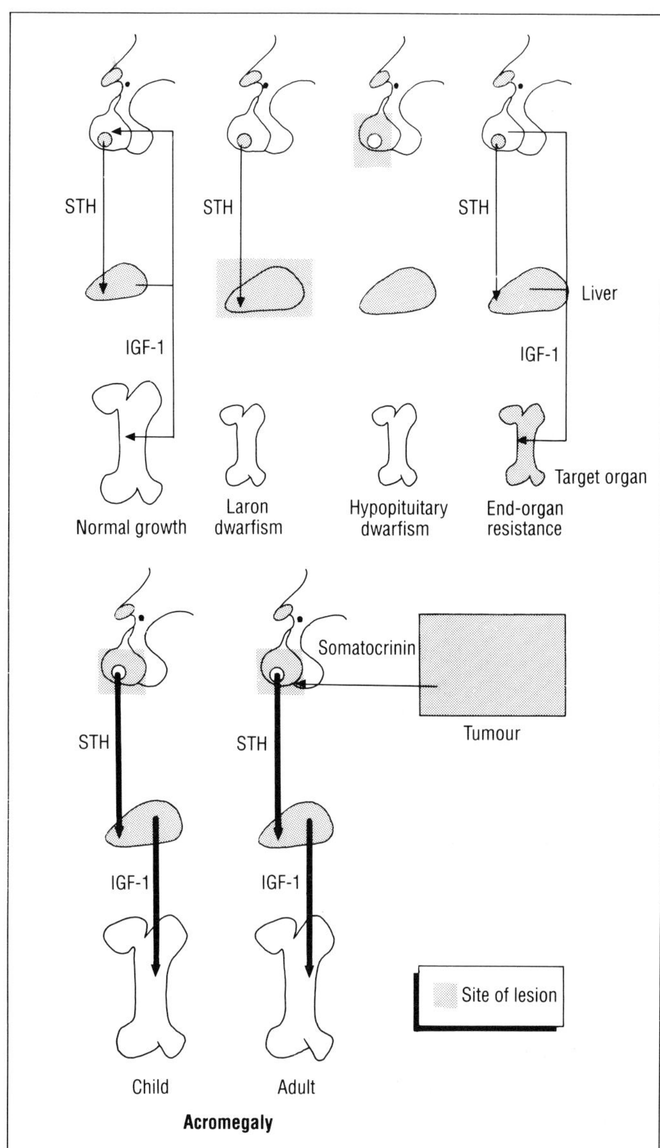

Fig. 46.2 Pathophysiology of somatotrophin secretion.

47 Endocrine–immune interactions

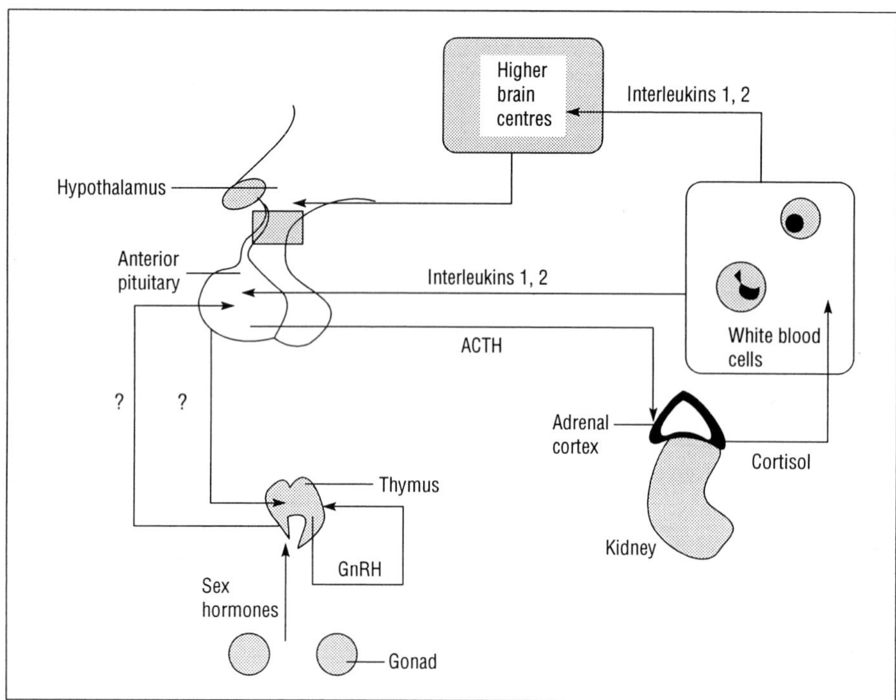

Fig. 47.1 Endocrine–immune interactions.

Evidence is growing that the endocrine and immune systems affect each other through hormones and other chemical messengers. Steroid hormones such as the glucocorticoids and the sex hormones have been known for years to have atrophic actions on the thymus, and glucocorticoids, such as dexamethasone and prednisolone, are routinely prescribed in rheumatoid arthritis and other autoimmune diseases to suppress immune function. Glucocorticoids induce apoptosis (programmed cell death) in cells of the immune system, and in some diseases, such as systemic lupus erythematosus (SLE), an autoimmune disease which primarily affects women, oestrogens are known to exacerbate the disease. In pregnancy, suppression of the immune system in the region of the site of implantation is essential if the blastocyst is not to be rejected by the host tissue (the endometrium). There are therefore strong grounds for suspecting that the two systems are intimately involved in each other's function in many ways.

THE CORTICOTROPHIN-RELEASING FACTOR/ ADRENOCORTICOTROPHIC HORMONE SYSTEM

The corticotrophin-releasing factor/adrenocorticotrophic hormone (CRF–ACTH) system affects and is affected by hormones and mediators of the immune system. In the CRF–ACTH system (see page 34), the hypothalamus produces CRF, which stimulates ACTH production, and ACTH promotes the release of adrenal steroids. It is now known that leukocytes (white blood cells) produce ACTH. Interestingly, leukocyte ACTH production is stimulated by a virus, Newcastle disease virus (NDV). *In vitro* experiments have shown that CRF stimulates expression of the pro-opiomelanocortin (POMC) gene (see page 35) in pituitary, spleen and thymocyte cells, and promotes ACTH release from all these cells. Furthermore, dexamethasone inhibits ACTH release from immune cells, suggesting that a negative-feedback neuroendocrine-type system exists in circulating white cells of the immune system.

The cytokines interleukin (IL) 1 and 2, which are released by activated macrophages and thymocyte (T) cells respectively, have a similar action to CRF in stimulating ACTH production and release from cells of the anterior pituitary gland and from lymphocytes. IL-1 and IL-2 receptors have been found on pituitary corticotrophs, suggesting that the cytokines may act as hormonal modulators of ACTH release from the pituitary.

The functional significance of an integrated immune–endocrine CRF–ACTH system is unclear at present, but the two may work together in, for example, responses to stress. Viral infections may trigger cortisol production in cells of the immune system, while environmental stresses such as cold or mental stress may cause cortisol secretion via the hypothalamus–pituitary–adrenal axis. CRF may be a physiological activator of the immune system, stimulating cytokine production, and possibly also stimulating natural killer (NK) cell activity. NK cells are large, granular lymphocytes which attack tumour cells.

THE THYMUS

The thymus is a lobed organ overlying the heart in the thorax. It is essential for the development of the fetus, and for differentiation and maturation of thymocytes which are released into the circulation. The thymus 'teaches' T cells to single out foreign antigens. After passage through the thymus, mature lymphocytes are competent as cytotoxic helpers or suppressors, that is, T cells which interact with each other or cells of the immune system, helping them to proliferate into antibody-producing plasma cells after their cognate antigen has entered the body.

Thymus atrophy. The thymus starts to atrophy after puberty in humans, and gradually becomes a fatty tissue. The sex hormones in physiological concentrations are atrophic to the thymus, as are stress and the adrenal corticosteroids. The thymus atrophies quite markedly during pregnancy. Even after removal of the gonads, the thymus continues to atrophy through life, and there may be an inbuilt programme of cell death or apoptosis in the ageing thymus.

Traditionally, it was thought that the thymus had no role in adult life, but it is now known that the adult thymus continues to secrete peptides into the peripheral circulation, and the thymus may therefore be a functioning endocrine gland throughout life.

Thymus hormones. The thymus epithelium produces and releases a number of peptides into the circulation. *Thymopoietin* is a peptide of 49 amino acids. *Thymulin* is a smaller peptide of 9 amino acids, and both thymopoietin and thymulin bind to T cells, and are involved in an as yet unknown way in T-cell differentiation. Both hormones bind to T-cell precursors, on which they induce differentiation antigens and the characteristic functions of a particular T-cell lineage. Another thymus family of peptide hormones, the *thymosins*, appears to mediate the conversion of immature prothymocytes into mature thymocytes. Thymus hormones are currently being tested for possible efficacy in certain immune deficiency syndromes. The thymus has also been found to produce the neuropeptide gonadotrophin-releasing hormone (GnRH), which has regenerative effects on the ageing thymus.

48 Steroidogenesis enzymes

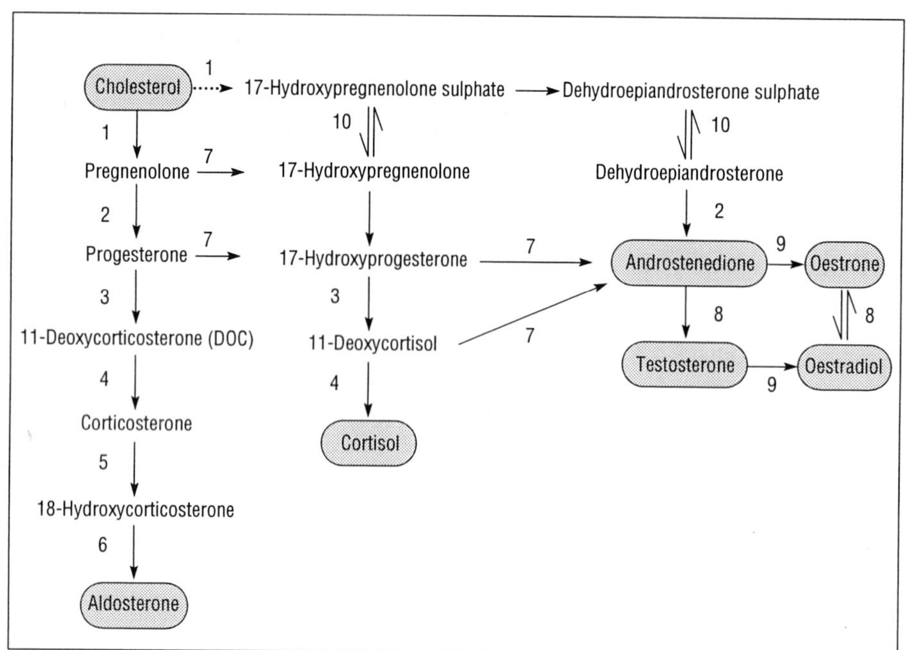

Fig. 48.1 Steroidogenesis summary.

ENZYMES

1 *Desmolase system* (20 and 22 hydroxylases and C20–22 desmolase activity): desmolase enzymes split double bonds, which become destabilized after the introduction of hydroxyl or ketone groups on adjacent carbon atoms.

2 *3-Beta-hydroxysteroid oxidoreductase/Delta$_{4-5}$ oxosteroid isomerase enzymes*: these enzymes are situated in the microsomes, use NAD^+ as a co-factor, and convert DHEA (dehydroepiandrosterone) and pregnenolone into androstenedione and progesterone respectively.

3 *21-Hydroxylase*: hydroxylases, also occasionally referred to in the literature as oxidases, are complex enzyme systems. Some are localized in the microsomes (C17, C21), and some in the mitochondria (C11, C18, C19, C20, C22). The general formula for the type of reaction they catalyse is $RH + \frac{1}{2}O_2 + NADPH \rightarrow ROH + NADP + H_2O$.

4 *11-Beta-hydroxylase.*

5 *18-Hydroxylase.*

6 *18-Hydroxysteroid oxidoreductase*: this enzyme, in the adrenal zona glomerulosa, converts 18-hydroxycorticosterone to aldosterone. The zona glomerulosa lacks 17-hydroxylase. Progesterone becomes hydroxylated at C21 and C11-beta, which produces corticosterone. This is followed by hydroxylation at C18, and oxidation of the alcohol moiety to an aldehyde, which yields aldosterone.

7 *C17–20 Desmolase.*

8 *17-Beta-hydroxysteroid oxidoreductase*: this enzyme is localized mainly in the ovary, placenta and testes, although it has also been found in erythrocytes (red blood cells), the kidney and liver.

9 *Aromatase*: the aromatase system consists of a C19 hydroxylase and a hydroxysteroid oxidoreductase. Testosterone and androstenedione are converted to oestradiol and oestrone, respectively, by aromatization of the A ring. Aromatization is the creation of an alternating double bond system in the six-membered ring, which confers what is called *resonance* to the ring, and gives it chemical stability. Initially, C19 is hydroxylated, followed by the oxidation and removal of a molecule of HCHO (formaldehyde).

10 *Sulphotransferase/sulphatase system*: this system consists of soluble enzymes, present mainly in the liver and placenta, although smaller quantities occur in the adrenal gland. The enzymes utilize sulphate moieties contained in the co-enzyme 3′-phosphate adenosine 5′-phosphosulphate (PAPS). In the adrenal gland, PAPS occurs mainly in the zona reticularis.

Further reading

Baulieu E-E and Kelly P.A. (eds.) (1990) *Hormones: From Molecules to Disease*. Chapman and Hall, New York.

Berne R.M. and Levy M.N. (eds.) (1990) *Principles of Physiology*. International student edition. Wolfe Publishers, London.

Edwards C.R.W. (ed.) (1986) *Endocrinology*. Heinemann, London.

Guyton A.C. (1991) *Textbook of Medical Physiology* (8th edn). W.B. Saunders, Philadelphia.

Hardy R.N. (1984) *Endocrine Physiology*. Edward Arnold, London.

Horwitz K.B. (ed.) (1993) Endocrine aspects of cancer. In *Endocrine Reviews and Monographs*. The Endocrine Society, Bethesda.

Lightman S.L. and Everitt B.J. (eds.) (1986) *Neuroendocrinology*. Blackwell Scientific Publications, Oxford.

O'Riordan J.L.H., Malan P.G. and Gould R.P. (eds.) (1984) *Essentials of Endocrinology*. Blackwell Scientific Publications, Oxford.

Parker M.G. (ed.) (1993) *Steroid Hormone Action*. IRL Press, Oxford.

Ross M.H., Reith E.J. and Romrell L.J. (1989) *Histology: A Text and Atlas* (2nd edn). Williams and Wilkins, Baltimore.

Snell R.S. (1987) *Clinical Neuroanatomy for Medical Students* (2nd edn). Little, Brown, Boston.

Wingard L.B., Brody T.M., Larner J. and Schwartz A. (1991) *Human Pharmacology*. International student edition. Wolfe Publishers, London.

Yen S.S.C. and Vale W.W. (eds.) (November 1989) Neuroendocrine control of reproduction. Proceedings of the symposium on neuroendocrine regulation of reproduction. Serono Symposia USA.

Glossary of terms

ablation surgical removal of tumours, gangrenous areas and damaged tissues
adipose tissue fat
aetiology cause (of a disease)
agonist ligand which elicits normal response
allosteric proteins changing conformation
AMP adenosine monophosphate
anion negatively charged ion, for example, PO_4^-
antigen substance capable of producing immune response
apical top, at apex
asymptotic without symptoms
avian pertaining to birds
axon cytoplasmic extension extending away from nerve cell body
beta-blocker substance blocking sympathetic beta-receptor
buccal mucosa inner mucosal lining of cheek or mouth
C-terminal acidic carboxyl group (COOH) end of peptide chain
carotinaemia vitamin A deficiency
catabolism breakdown
catalyse act as a catalyst
catalyst unchanged substance enabling a chemical reaction
catecholamines amine derivatives of 2-hydroxyphenol (catechol)
cation positively charged ion, for example, Na^+
civet member of feline family
clitoris female erectile organ homologous with penis
colloid dispersion of high molecular weight substance in fluid
congenital condition or defect present from birth
cortex outer layer of organ or structure
cytoplasm intracellular living part of cell outside nucleus
de novo new
dermopathy disease of skin
dimerization combination of two protein molecules
diploid cell has two sets of chromosomes
endocrine gland ductless gland
endogenous originating inside body
endoplasmic intracellular membrane system
epinephrine US terminology for adrenaline
epithelium sheets of cells lining surfaces
euthyroid clinically normal thyroid function
exocytosis cellular secretion of packaged molecules
exogenous originating outside body
fibroblasts flattened, irregular connective tissue cells
follicle group of cells in functional unit, for example, thyroid, ovary
ganglion mass of nerve cell bodies
gender self-perceived sex
genitalia reproductive organs
genotype genetic make-up of the organism
gestation pregnancy, intra-uterine period for fetus
globulin class of proteins soluble in weak salt solutions
gluconeogenesis new synthesis of glucose
glycogen polysaccharide storage form of glucose
glycogenolysis glycogen breakdown
glycosylation adding oligosaccharide side chains to proteins
GTP guanosine triphosphate
haploid cell has one set of chromosomes
homeostasis internal control of internal environment
homeotherm 'warm blooded', internal temperature control
homology structural resemblance
hydrophilic water-attracting
hydrophobic water-repellent, uncharged
hypertension clinically diagnosed high blood pressure
hypothermia clinically significant, low body temperature
iatrogenic disease-producing prescription
idiopathic unknown cause
in vivo in the living body
in vitro outside the living body, 'in glass'
insomnia lack of sleep, inability to fall asleep
intercalate insert into (usually into DNA)
ischaemia localized tissue death through oxygen lack
karyotype paired arrangement of chromosome set ranked in size
kinase enzyme transferring inorganic PO_4^- from adenosine triphosphate (ATP) to acceptor
labia lips, lip–lip structure, here referring to vulva
ligand one molecule that binds reversibly to another
lyse break-up, usually referring to cell disruption
medulla inner or central layer of organ or structure
meiosis nuclear division from diploid to haploid
metabolism integration of biochemical reactions in the body
microgram 10^{-6}g
mitochondria intracellular organelles producing energy
mitosis cell division with retention of diploid
muscarinic acetylcholine receptor blocked by muscarine
myelinogenesis synthesis of nerve myelin sheath
N-terminals basic NH_2 end of peptide chain
nicotinic acetylcholine receptor stimulated by nicotine
nona- nine
norepinephrine US terminology for noradrenaline
octa- eight
olfactory pertaining to sense of smell
oligosaccharides linked reducing sugars (or monosaccharides)
oscillator mechanism pre-set to return to a value if perturbed
osteoclast bone-destroying multinucleate cell
penis erectile male reproductive organ
phenotype visible or measurable characteristics of organism
poikilotherm 'cold-blooded', body temperature, depends on environment
precursor parent substance
primordial primitive
progestational eliciting progesterone-like responses
proteolysis breakdown of protein
transcription copying of DNA to form complementary RNA
transducer converter of sensory input to another energy form
translation production of peptide according to mRNA coding

trimester defined 3-month period of pregnancy
trophic causing growth
ultimobranchial gland calcitonin-producing avian gland
vulva mammalian external genitalia
zona glomerulosa outer layer of adrenal cortex

SOURCES

Lawrence E. (1989) *Henderson's Dictionary of Biological Terms* (10th edn). Longman Scientific and Technical, Essex

Concise Medical Dictionary (3rd edn) (1987). Oxford University Press, Oxford

Index